ARLENE PHILLIPS'
KEEP
IN
SHAPE
SYSTEM

ARLENE PHILLIPS'

KEEP IN SHAPE SYSTEM

by Arlene Phillips

Ferroway Press

Published by
Fanfare books
46 South Molton Street
London W1Y 1HE

ISBN: 0 – 86370 – 000 – 4

© FANFARE BOOKS 1985

Reprinted 1985

Produced by
Michael Balfour Ltd
3 Wedgwood Mews
Greek Street
London W1V 5LW

Executive Producer	Iain Burton
Editor-in-Chief	Michael Balfour
Project Co-ordinator	Belinda Davies
Designers	Field Wylie & Company
Photographer	Mike Owen
Make-up and Hair	Elenka
Leotards and Tights	Carita House
Typesetting	Project Reprographics Ltd
Printed	The Bath Press, Avon

KISS (Keep In Shape System) is a trademark of Ferroway Ltd, London

Contents

Warm thanks to Kathy Burke who has worked closely with me on the KISS concept. Like me, Kathy believes that dancing and exercise are for everyone. She started dancing late—at 19—and became totally dedicated, studying and training. After working with me for 10 years, she is now a successful teacher and choreographer in her own right. We're still great friends, enjoy working together and are currently involved in several exciting new projects.

Introduction

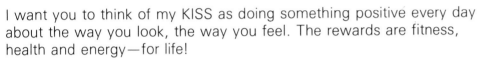

Do you want to get your body in super-shape, tuned in to high-energy? Start by reading right through this book. But in fact it is what happens next that really matters! If you neatly put it away on a bookshelf, we're all wasting our time ... this book is to read and then 'do'. And the 'doing' is learning a system of exercises designed to work every part of your body, with the plus of aerobercises to rev-up your energy. These are backed up with an eating plan for maximum health and vitality, and a positive strategy to combat the stress that can rob you of your health as well as sapping your energy.

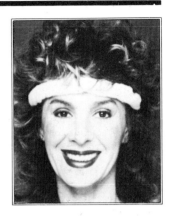

I want you to think of my KISS as doing something positive every day about the way you look, the way you feel. The rewards are fitness, health and energy—for life!

I want you to work your body, but not punish it; work *with* your body and not against it. So be realistic. If you have not exercised in years start slowly—stay with the Warm-Up (Chapter 1) until you're doing it without any strain, then move on gradually—you'll get there! Too much, too soon and you'll give up.

You'll be amazed at how much your body improves in shape and stamina. I never get tired of seeing it happen in my classes: watching flab disappear, watching waists and thighs re-appear. After just a few months of classes, you can look years younger, experience new highs of energy, and be in better shape than you ever thought possible.

I've developed my Keep In Shape System (KISS) over 16 years of teaching exercise and dance; and years of study before that. In fact, I went to my first dance class when I was 2. I loved it right from the start, knowing it was what I wanted to do. At nine I joined the Muriel Tweedy School of Ballet in Manchester and graduated into teaching there. At 21 I was stuck for an idea as to how to spend my summer holidays. Miss Tweedy suggested I go to London and try some ballet classes at a new dance centre. The first thing I saw there was an advertisement for American jazz dancing classes. I was intrigued, skipped the ballet class, went to the jazz, and after just one lesson I was hooked! I decided right there and then to stay in London and study American jazz dancing.

I took some strange jobs, like shaking mothballs out of army surplus clothes, just to pay for tuition for two years with teacher Molly Molloy. I became one of her teachers and got more and more interested in choreography. My first real piece of choreography was for an ice cream commercial, starring a cow! Luckily for me it was directed by Ridley Scott, and the commercial was a big success. That led to me choreographing just about any commercial with dance in it, both here and in the USA.

There was a rumble of interest in the routines I did for Love Machine on *The Benny Hill Show*. That rumble became more like an explosion after Hot Gossip made their TV debut! People thought Gossip were an overnight success, but not at all. I formed Hot Gossip seven years ago; its members came from my students, the name came from a friend who was always ringing up with what he called ''the latest hot gossip''

My three-year-old daughter Alana was born into dancing. Two days before her birth I was rehearsing dance sequences for the film *Can't Stop the Music*; a week later I was back at work filming them and Alana came too. She continued to travel with me on the films that followed: *The Fan* in New York when she was one; *Annie* in New York and Los Angeles when she was two, and then to Bradford with the Monty Python film when she was three.

Fortunately I keep busy with choreography for film and stage musicals and with TV work, but I would never give up teaching exercise and dance classes. I have worked with hundreds of well-known people, but the ones I enjoy are those who really work hard. It is a pleasure to teach Pamela Stephenson, Lulu, Lauren Bacall, Stefanie Powers and Olivia Newton-John and many others. And, if you've watched Hot

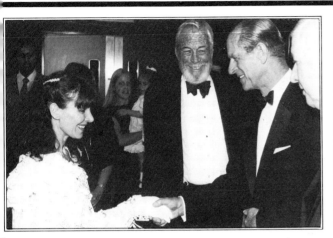 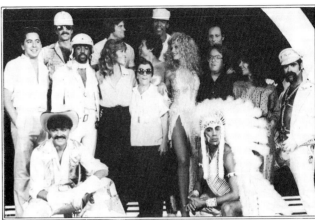

Gossip, you'll know my style of dance and movement does not exclude men. In fact, David Essex was the first person to give Hot Gossip their big break, even before Kenny Everett. Since then I have worked with many other male stars, including Wayne Sleep and Michael Crawford.

I call my programme 'stretch out and dance', because to me exercise and dance are so closely linked. Every dance class starts with exercise—it is essential. And what I teach you in this book is how to exercise correctly, and then get you moving the Hot Gossip way.

My life is busy; sometimes it is work 12 hours a day and longer for seven days a week. People are always asking me where all the energy comes from and how I stay in shape. I've written this book to answer that question! I do have natural high energy, but I know that it is my exercises that keep it high, and give me stamina. Like millions of people, I'm not naturally slim; I have to work at it through exercise, dance and diet. You cannot change your skeleton and body type. If you have short legs, broad hips and a high proportion of body fat to muscle (a natural endomorph), there is no point in yearning to be an all-angles, lean, long-limbed ectomorph. Recognise your body type and then work to get your body in its own best possible shape. If you have not exercised seriously before, your body has a lot more potential than you realise!

Good body shape depends on the holding force of the muscles. To do their work, the muscles have to be exercise-fit. All muscles start out long and lean, as muscles must be. But if you don't exercise they become short and bulging with the fat that forms inside the muscle. In this state, the muscles cannot do their job properly, the sag sets in and the flab takes hold. The combination of the stretching exercises and the fat-burning aerobercises will put that right.

When you start to exercise, you will become body-conscious; you stand tall and right away your sad, crumpled fat look starts to go! If you exercise regularly, you can increase the rate at which you burn calories. That means you don't have to reduce your intake so drastically as before and the weight you lose will stay lost. On its own dieting may drive the pounds away, but it can do nothing about the condition of your muscles. Without exercise, dieters go from fat and flabby to thin and flabby, which is not very attractive.

Exercise promotes good circulation, builds up the efficiency of heart and lungs, controls the appetite, and keeps the muscles and joints in good working order. It will increase your resistance to illness and generate energy to help you sail through hard work and hard play.

Convinced? Before you even get one foot into the leotard, get the exercise-killers out of the way! First, there's the totally wrong idea that exercise has to hurt to be doing you good. If an exercise hurts, you must stop doing it right away. More dangerous still is the very Californian, over-aerobic idea that you have to work through the pain to some new level of super-exercising. That doesn't make sense. It's a contradiction of the whole idea of aerobic, which is literally, exercising "with air". If you go on for too long, you'll be gasping for air, hyperventilating, feeling dizzy and sick, and your heart will be pounding in your head. Does that sound healthy? The aerobercises in Chapter 3 are going to do great things for you, but you *must* build up gradually; monitor your pulse and assess your own fitness as described in the chapter.

If you are in a hurry to get fit, making the exercises tougher won't help, but doing them more often will. The fastest way to get fit is to proceed with caution:

* Work at your own pace. You are not a failure if the exercise asks for 10 repetitions and you do 2. Congratulate yourself on the 2 you've done. You will get to 10 sooner than you think!

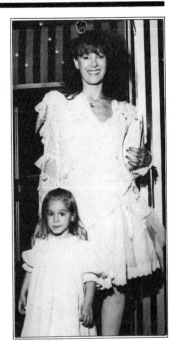

* Work hard, but don't become obsessive about exercise; it's there to get you looking good and feeling great, so that you can really *live* your life. Exercise isn't meant to dominate your life. And it can happen. I have known a few people become so obsessed with getting through their marathon exercise class that nothing else matters. They give up sex, they give up their family life—nothing else seems to matter.

* Read through my instructions and have a good look at the photographs *before* you start on any part of the exercise programmes.

Ready? Then turn to 'Warm-Up'. I try to do this every single morning—simply because it puts me in a higher gear for the rest of the day. Try it—it will work for you, too! And this is just the beginning of a *total* health and beauty adventure, because my KISS gives you a *whole* approach to your body. How to diet, how to look good (and therefore feel even better!) and how to relax are so important and you will find careful and valuable advice in Chapter 5, 6 and 7. Good wishes for a better life!

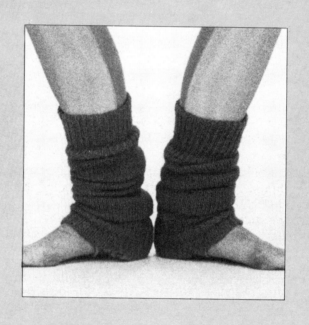

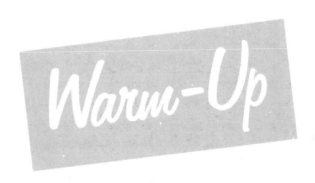

1

Warm-Up

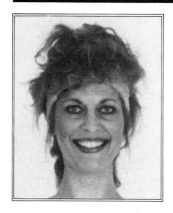

Gillian Elvins takes you through the Warm-Up. She's facing 40 and looking fabulous. These days she is mostly a mum, with occasional modelling jobs. She has two children; Alexandra, 7 and Sasha, 11, and they live near Godalming in Surrey. Gillian exercises of course to keep supple and slim. Like everybody else, she sometimes over-eats and puts on a couple of pounds; she always takes extra exercise until her weight is back to normal again.

R eady to start? Good. You should begin every exercise routine with a warm-up, and it is dangerous not to. Dancers and athletes always warm up. It loosens and lengthens the muscles and makes the joints more flexible. The exercises in this chapter will get the circulation going, carrying good supplies of oxygen and blood to the muscles so that they can be worked harder. Don't ever be tempted to skip the warm-up; you could end up straining or even tearing a muscle or ligament—bringing your fitness campaign to a crashing and painful halt. Remember the following points.

1. It is important to keep warm as you exercise. If you're in an ice-cold room, your muscles will tighten, bringing a danger of cramp, soreness and strain. Make sure the room is warm—if you're in any doubt, put on a tracksuit and leg warmers.

2. It is dangerous to wear tight clothing as it hampers circulation. Make sure you are wearing something that allows you to move easily; a leotard or tracksuit is ideal.

3. You don't need a special exercise mat; a carpet is fine.

4. Don't exercise after a heavy meal; wait at least two hours. Just after a meal more blood is diverted to the stomach, not to the muscles that need extra supplies when you exercise.

5. Remember to breathe! Lots of people hold their breath when they are new to exercise.

Warm-Up

You need full breathing to get oxygen into your bloodstream and remove the toxins.

6. Study the following photographs before you start. Use a mirror to check your positions as you work—especially at first. If you are a beginner, you won't be able to do the exercises as well as the women in the photographs—but in time you *will!* The only difference is that they have had lots of practice.

7. Try to do the exercises really well, but do *not* strain yourself. Push yourself a little bit further than you think you can go, but always listen to your body. Get to know the good feeling of a muscle that's being stretched. It is quite different from pain. If you feel pain stop at once, however simple the exercise you're doing.

8. If it is a long time since you did any exercise, you're probably going to feel stiff for a day or two afterwards. Look on this as a good sign. It means that unused muscles are back in action again—just what we want! Your beautiful new body is starting to take shape.

This Warm-Up is designed to wake up your body. That is why I use it as my early morning routine. Then I know that it will help me keep up my energy during the day. You may say you don't even have one minute to spare in the morning rush. But try it, you'll find it speeds you up, gets you really moving—so you're saving that time constantly throughout the day.

In the evenings, I do the Warm-Up again before going on to the rest of the exercise programme. I like to work through KISS at the end of a hard day, as I find that it really gives me an energy boost to enjoy the evening.

How often should you exercise? I think everybody should do the Warm-Up every day of their lives! Then it's up to you. You know how fit you want to be and how fast. But don't rush it. If you are very out of condition when you start, it's an excellent plan to do the Warm-Up once a day at first, and, after a few weeks, twice a day. You'll feel yourself getting more supple and more strong. Then you'll know that it's time to move on to the rest of KISS

You might enjoy exercising with friends. But please, never compete. There is a right speed and intensity for your work and only you can monitor that. Start by setting aside just 10 minutes a day. You'll soon notice how much better you look and feel—how your body is starting to get into shape! Let's exercise…

Warm-Up

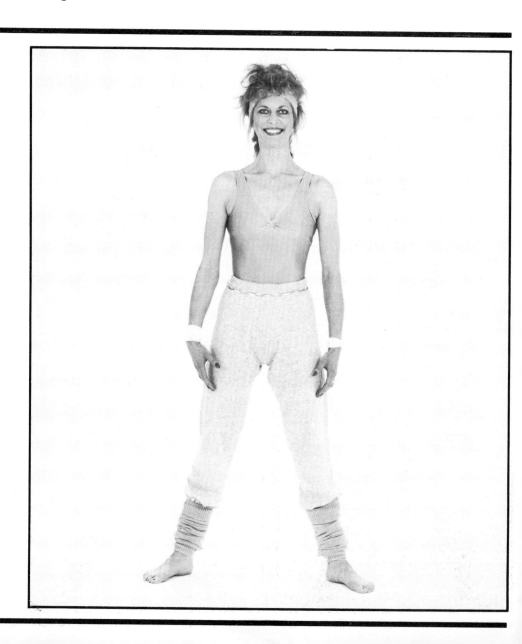

Warm-Up

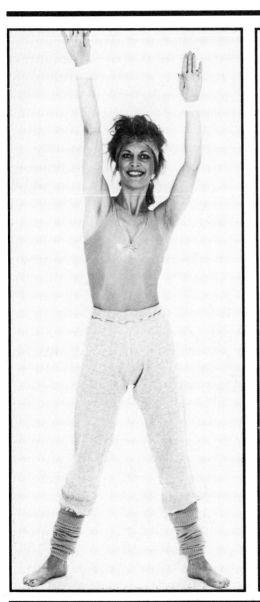

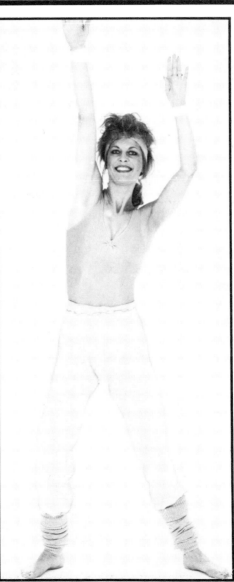

Starting position: Stand with your feet apart and pointing slightly outwards. Raise both arms above your head with the palms facing frontwards.

Breathing: Steadily throughout.

1. Stretch up with your right hand, aiming for the ceiling. Feel your ribs lifting up off your hips. Reach with left hand, then right, left.

2. This time, as you reach up with your right hand, bend your right knee (keep it directly over the right foot). Now with left hand and left knee. Repeat 1 and 2 three times altogether.

3. Relax your arms down to your sides and up again. Now repeat entire exercise four times.

Watchpoints: Try to make the upwards stretch go further each time and check your standing position: stomach should be pulled in and tail tucked under.

Benefits: Designed to start working on your waist—and give you a wide-awake feeling.

Warm-Up

EXERCISE TWO

Starting position: Stand with your feet apart and turned out. Make sure your legs are straight. Let your right hand rest on right thigh with left arm out at shoulder level.

Breathing: Out as you push to the side, in as you come up.

1. Bend to the right and reach over with your left arm. Feel that stretch and go on for a count of four. Come back up slowly.

2. With left hand resting on left thigh and right arm out at shoulder level, bend to the left, bringing the right arm over. Do four stretches to the side then come up slowly.

3. Repeat sixteen times in all, stretching to the count of four, getting a little further over each time.

Watchpoints: Keep your legs straight; check that your stomach is pulled in tight, and you bend directly to the side.

Benefits: Muscles are being loosened all down sides of body, and waistline is being improved.

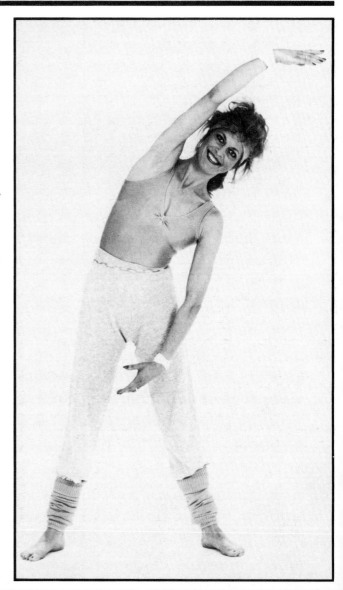

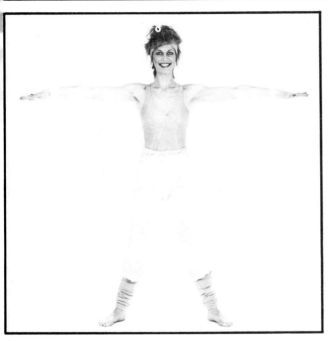 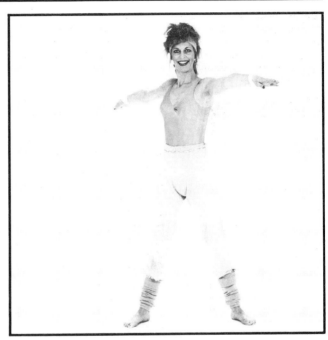

Starting position: Stand with your feet apart and in a comfortable position. Make sure legs are straight. Hold arms out at shoulder level.

Breathing: In on the swing and out on the wrap.

1. Using lots of energy, swing arms across the body to the right and wrap round. Follow through with upper part of the body. Swing back through starting position and continue the wrap to the left.

2. Do the swing six times more, alternating right and left.

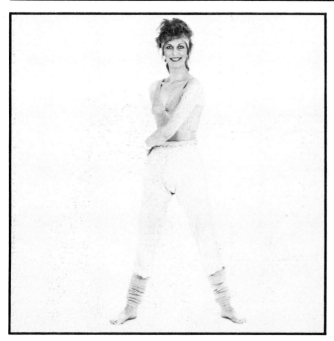

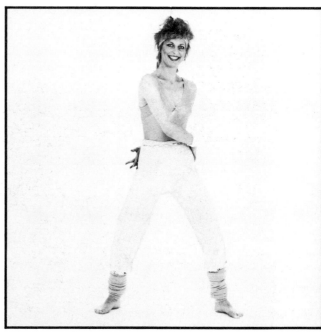

3. Now, as you swing and wrap, bend your knees. Straighten your knees as you unwrap. Do this eight times in all, swinging right and left alternately.

Watchpoints: To benefit from this exercise, your arms must swing through a straight line. Make sure your knees stay over your feet when legs bend. Make sure arms are working together, not separately.

Benefits: Revs up the circulation and begins to tone the body.

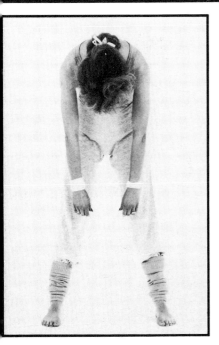

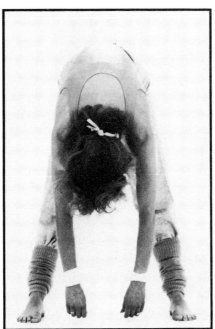

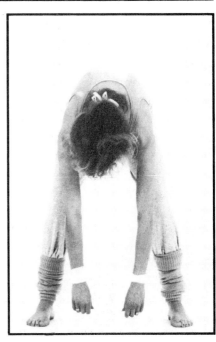

Starting position: Stand with your feet apart and parallel.

Breathing: Out as you relax forward, and in as you come up.

1. Relax your neck and let your head roll down, keeping chin as close as possible to your chest, come up very slowly. Repeat.

2. This time as you go down bend your knees. Go down really low and get your head close to the floor. Straighten knees and roll up again. Repeat.

Watchpoints: Take this one very easily. If you feel any pain in spine—stop, relax and try again, not going so far down.

Benefits: The spine is stretched ready for the hard work to come.

Warm-Up

EXERCISE FIVE

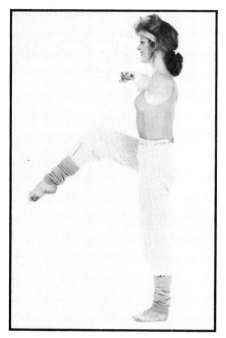 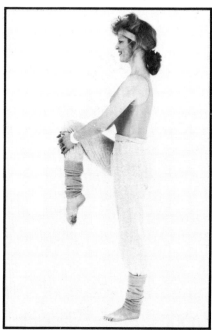 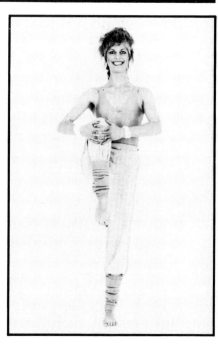

Starting position: Stand with your feet slightly apart and parallel (facing front). Arms held out to the side.

Breathing: Steadily throughout.

1. Keeping the left leg perfectly still, swing the right leg up in front of you, keeping the knee relaxed. Swing down to starting position, swing left leg up. Continue until you have done sixteen in all.

2. This time, as you swing the right leg up in front of you, catch hold of it with both hands and pull the knee right into the chest. Pull in four times. Lower leg. Repeat with the left leg. Repeat right, left right, left right, left.

Watchpoints: Make sure that the supporting leg stays straight. Try to get knee closer and closer to chest each time. Don't hunch shoulders.

Benefits: Good for thighs and bottom.

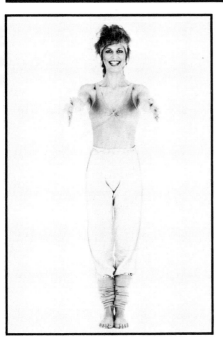 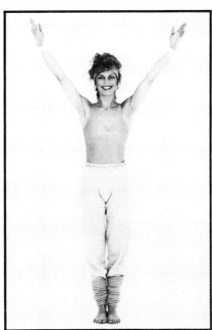 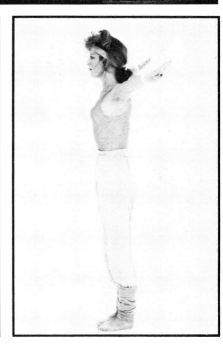

Starting position: Stand with the feet together and make sure that the spine is straight. Arms out at shoulder level.

Breathing: Naturally throughout.

1. Make huge backward circles with both arms eight times.

2. Change to forward circles and do eight of these.

3. Do eight more in each direction.

4. Make it even more energetic; as you circle your arms, jump in the air at the same time, eight times for the backward circles; eight more times for the forward circles. Try to repeat again.

Watchpoints: Make sure the circles are huge.

Benefits: This will really get the blood circulating. Now you'll be warmed up—ready for anything (well, almost!)

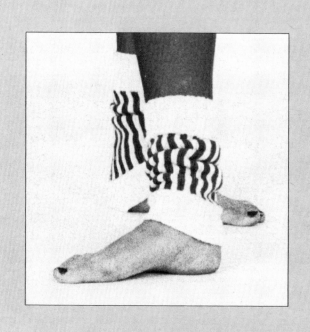

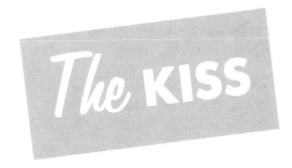

The KISS

2

The KISS

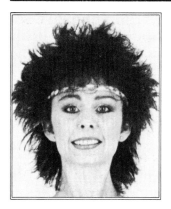

Bonita Bryg is 32 and looks about half that. She is the liveliest person I know and buzzes with energy. And where does all that energy come from? She puts it down to lots of dancing and eating masses of fresh vegetables, bread and yogurt every day – with a vitamin pill as insurance (especially when work means she can't stop for regular meal breaks). Bonny is one of those enviable people who worry about keeping their weight **up**, so she always eats good food, when she needs extra calories!

N ow you've done the Warm-Up, you're ready to get to work shaping your body—and KISS is designed to do just that. Being in good shape is where beauty and health really begin. A body that sags and bulges all over the place isn't going to make you feel good about yourself but, just as important, it's a health hazard.

Think about your stomach. If you don't exercise, the muscles are going to go slack. Your stomach will bulge out; you'll be at risk from digestive problems and from low back pain as the abdominal muscles can no longer do their job. A healthy back is one that is properly aligned, and this depends on the sinews, supported by the abdominal muscles, holding the pelvis where it belongs.

A body that is not exercised loses its strength and flexibility, and nothing works as well as it should! You simply get tired out very quickly, just by day-to-day living.

KISS is designed to counteract this by working your body *all over*. That is why it is important to work right through the following sequences. Even if you're mostly interested in getting rid of the flab on your thighs, don't rush to that section. You won't be getting the maximum benefits. It is regular exercise that works, so start by doing the KISS three times a week, and work up to five times.

The only time you shouldn't exercise is when you're ill. Even if you have a simple cold, your body needs its resources to fight the infection. But exercise will help you resist infections.

The exercises are planned to be safe to do without a teacher to keep an eye on you. But that means doing the exercises as shown in the pictures. Don't vary them. For instance, my sit-ups are all done from a bent knee position. This is deliberate, so please don't change it to flat leg position. Sitting up from that position can put too much strain on the back, especially if you're starting on my exercise system with weak stomach muscles.

There are some benefits you'll get from KISS that you might not be expecting. It is an effective depression fighter. When you exercise, certain chemicals are released into the blood which act as natural anti-depressants. Of course, exercise won't make problems go away, but it will make you more able to face up to them. Tension and anxiety are helped, too. When you're over-anxious, lactic acid levels in the blood shoot up. Exercise is an effective way of lowering those levels.

As you work through the exercises, try to keep the action smooth and easy; don't jerk, don't rush. Keep going at your own speed. If you are in a hurry to get fit, exercise more frequently, don't push yourself to do the exercises harder than your body is ready for.

It's important that your body is in the right position before you start. Stand in front of the mirror and have a good look:

1. Weight should be centred, you shouldn't be leaning forwards or backwards.
2. Is your chin at a perfect right angle to your throat? If not stretch up from the back of the neck and realign it.
3. Do your shoulders look hunched up? Pull them up and let them fall loosely down so that you can feel them relax.
4. Make sure hips are level and abdomen is lifted and pulled in.
5. Bottom should be neatly tucked under rather than clenched.
6. Make sure ankles are not sagging outwards or inwards.
7. The overall impression should be easy; look for any special points of tension and unknot them.

Now you're standing properly you're ready for the following five sets of exercise. I have called them Stretch, Toning-up, Top Half, On The Floor and Workout. Work well; some of it's going to be tough! But you'll love the results as your body gets firm and shapely.

The KISS

EXERCISE ONE

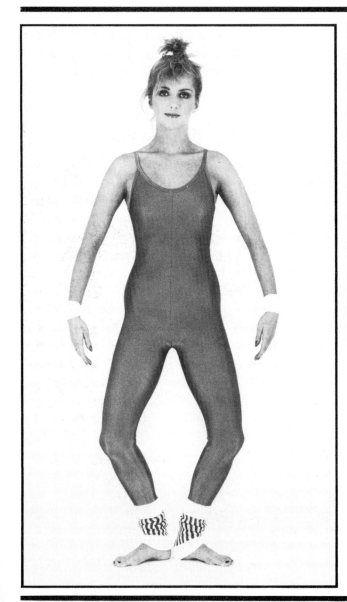

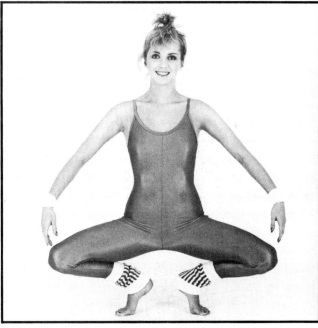

Starting position: Stand with your heels together and toes turned out; pull backs of your legs together and keep your arms relaxed by your side.

Breathing: Out on the way down, in on the way up.

1. Bend both knees, keeping them directly over the toes. Heels must stay together and the feet should stay on the floor. Come up again and repeat.

2. Bend the knees again. This time go down low, letting the heels come slowly up off the floor. As you come up again, put the heels down as soon as you can.

EXERCISE ONE

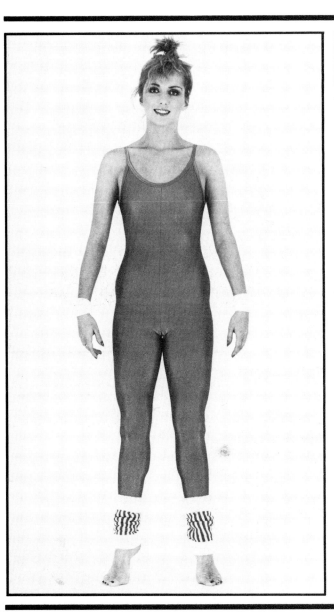

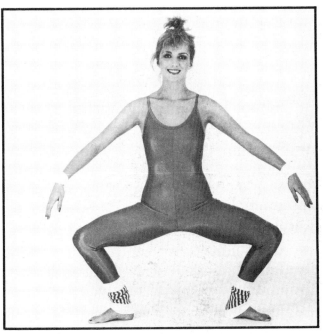

3. Do two more bends keeping your heels on the floor and then rise up on to the balls of your feet and hold for a count of eight. Keep the knees straight.

4. Repeat entire sequence.

5. Go through 1 to 4 again, but this time start with the legs wide apart and toes pointing out as much as you can. Keep your heels on the ground all the time.

Watchpoints: You may find it easier to hold on to a chair for this exercise—until your legs become strong. Try to keep your body as upright as possible, not making a sitting shape.

Benefits: Excellent for the thighs.

The **KISS**

EXERCISE TWO

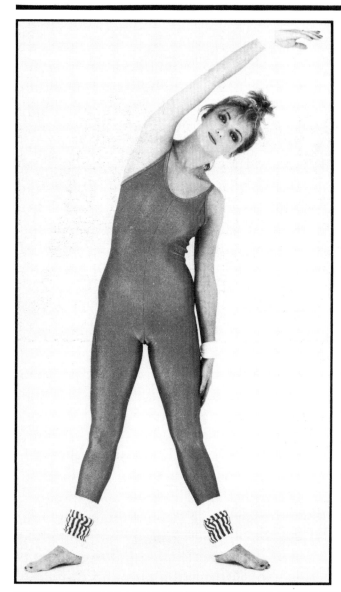

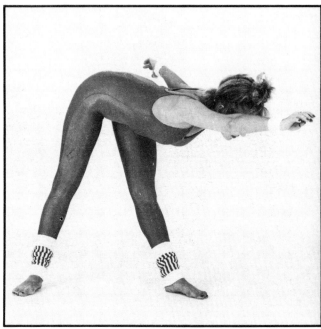

Starting position: Stand with your feet apart and turned out. Check that back is straight, stomach and tail tucked in.

Breathing: Naturally throughout.

1. Bend to the right, reaching over with the left arm. Come up again and then bend to the left, bringing the right arm over.

2. Stretch forward to the right corner of the room with the left arm. Come up and stretch to the left corner of the room with the right arm.

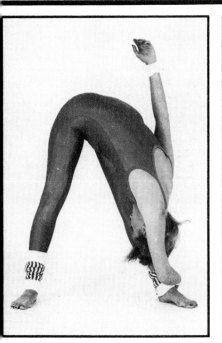

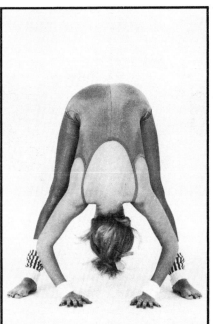

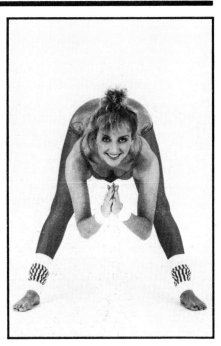

3. Relax with right hand down to left foot, trying to get your head on to your knee. Come back up and repeat with left hand down to right foot.

4. Relax forward until arms touch the floor. Clap the hands, touch the floor, clap the hands. Come back up to the starting position and repeat whole sequence four times.

Watchpoints: Don't worry if you can't get head down as far as Jane does. In time you will.

Benefits: A general conditioning exercise—good "all-rounder".

The KISS

EXERCISE THREE

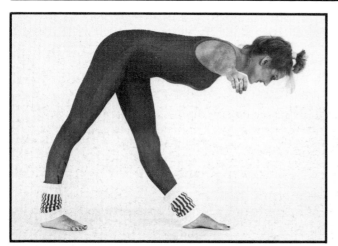

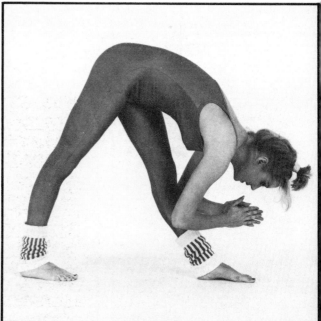

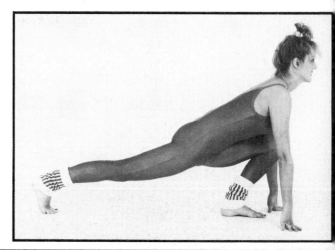

Starting position: Face the side with your feet wide apart and right foot in front of left. Hold arms out to side at shoulder level.

Breathing: Easily, and don't strain.

1. Gently bounce forward, with a flat back, four times.

2. Relax forward, dropping head down towards the front foot. Touch the floor, clap the hands, touch the floor, clap the hands. Do the whole thing four times.

3. Put both hands on the floor. Bend the front knee and let the back heel come off the floor, stretching out the back leg. Bounce there four times keeping the back straight.

4. As you come up, lower the back heel and reach forward with the arms. Stand up facing front and bringing arms up above head. Turn to face other side, lowering arms.

5. Repeat the entire sequence four times in all.

Watchpoints: On first half of the exercise make sure the weight is evenly distributed on both legs.

Benefits: Works front and back of thighs. Stretches lower spine and hips.

Far Right:
The best class is when I can really mix it! Pictured here – a couple of the dancers from 'Hot Gossip', beginners and regular students like Gillian.

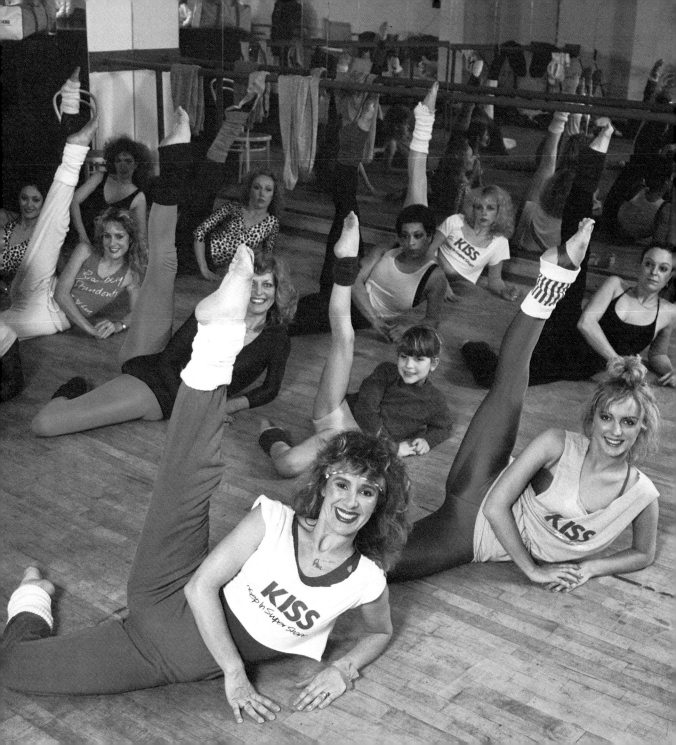

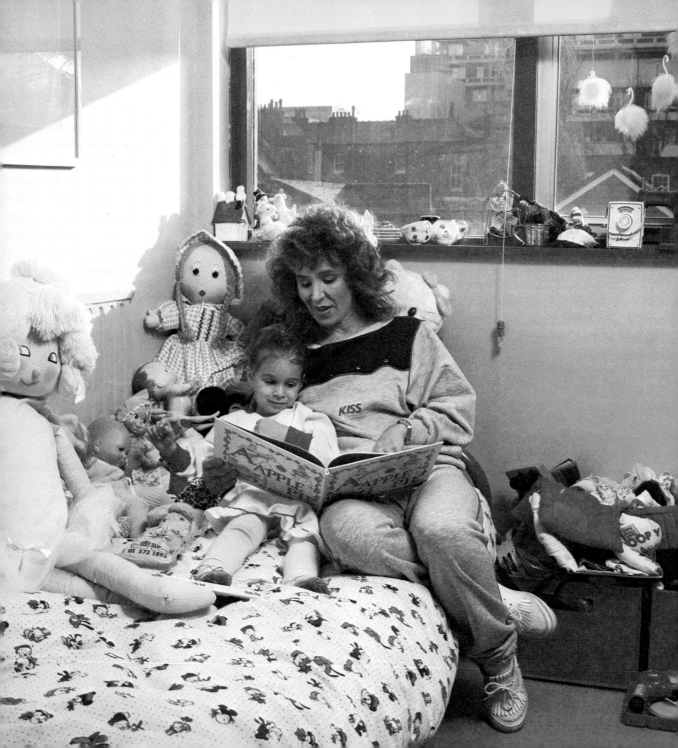

EXERCISE FOUR

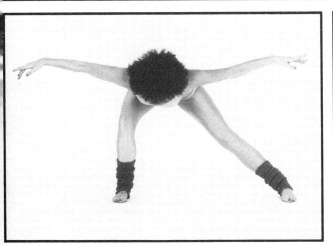

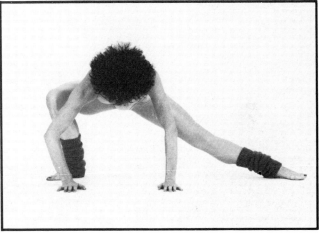

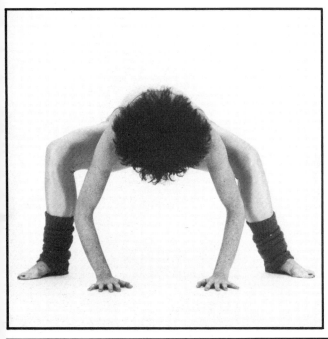

Starting position: Stand with legs wide apart, feet and legs both turned out. Check spine is straight, bottom and stomach tucked in. Hold arms out at shoulder level.

Breathing: Gently throughout.

1. Stretch forward with flat back. Lunge, bending the right knee and keeping arms at shoulder level. Gently bounce three times. Now lunge to left and bounce three times.

2. Drop down to floor by bending the right knee. Put your hands flat on the floor and pointing forward. Check that right knee is over toes and left knee is facing the ceiling. Bounce three times.

3. Start transferring your weight by putting your left heel on the floor and then walking through with your hands until left knee is over toes and right knee is facing ceiling—position reversed. Bounce there three times.

4. Repeat the whole sequence.

Watchpoints: Exercise gently at first, then try to increase the stretch.

Benefits: Works on legs and thighs and firms bottom.

Far Left:
Coming home to Alana after a hard day's work is magic! She tells me about her day, then we share a bedtime story. I enjoy it as much as she does . . .

The KISS

TONING-UP—EXERCISE ONE (This exercise is not included on the KISS album)

Starting position: Feet together and pointing forwards. Check that stomach is pulled in. Let arms rest naturally by your sides.

Breathing: Steadily all the way through.

1. Bend the knees then straighten them and rise up on to the balls of the feet; lower. Repeat four times slowly, then sixteen times very fast!

2. Bend the knees and, keeping them bent, rise up on to balls of feet. Ankles and knees should be together and back straight. Still on balls of feet, straighten knees and slowly lower heels. Do this four times slowly; then eight times fast.

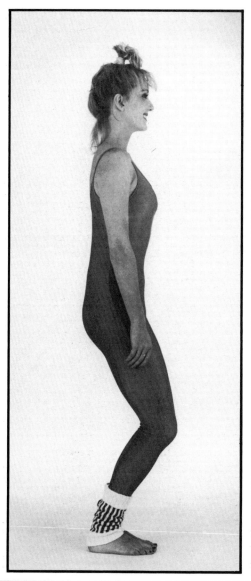
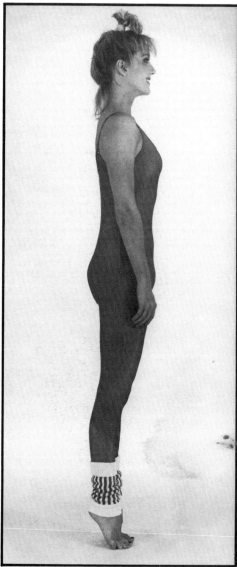

EXERCISE TWO

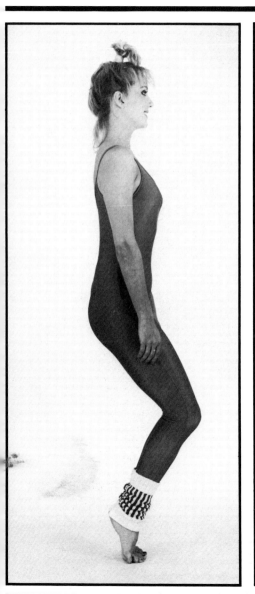

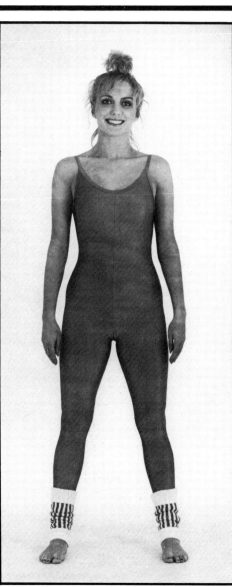

3. Rise up on balls of feet, bend the knees and lower the heels. Straighten knees. Do this four times slowly and then eight times fast.

4. Repeat the exercise all the way through, but this time have your feet apart and parallel.

Watchpoints: Try to squeeze inner thighs together for added strength.

Benefits: Ankles, knees, calves and thighs.

The KISS

EXERCISE TWO (This exercise is not included on the KISS album)

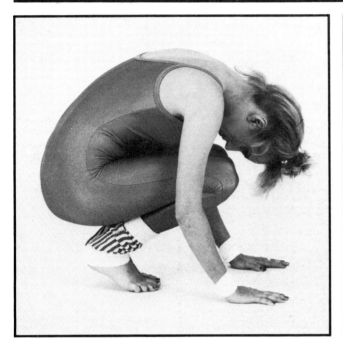 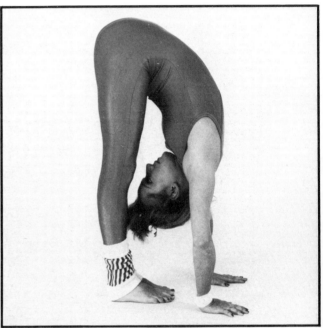

Starting position: Stand tall with feet together and arms by your side.

Breathing: Steadily throughout.

1. Drop down to the floor, bending both knees and letting the heels come up off the floor. Rest hands flat on the floor.

2. Do easy bounces, pressing the inner thighs, the ankles and knees together as much as possible.

3. Lower the heels to the floor, straighten both knees, try to keep hands flat on floor and head close to knees as you relax forward.

4. Repeat all the way through four times. Then repeat eight times but only bounce twice before straightening up; this makes it faster.

Watchpoints: It takes lots of practice to get in a perfect position; don't worry, just keep on working. Don't push heels up high on the bounce.

Benefits: Legs will firm up, thighs and calves will become shapelier.

The KISS

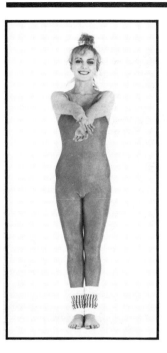

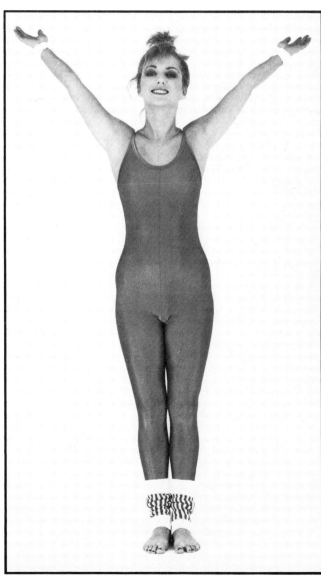

Starting position: Stand with feet together and facing front. Arms should be held out in front with palms facing the ceiling.

Breathing: Inhale and exhale deeply.

1. Swing the arms out as wide as you can, keeping the palms facing the ceiling. Then close again. Do this sixteen times.

Watchpoints: Each time get that swing wider. If it's not wide, it won't work.

Benefits: Starts the work of firming the muscles that support the bust.

The KISS

EXERCISE TWO

Starting position: Stand with the feet together and facing front. Stretch arms in front with palms facing the ceiling.

Breathing: Steadily throughout.

1. Open your arms just a little way and then bring them in again in a fast chopping movement, trying to make little fingers touch as you beat sides of hands together.

2. Repeat the chops as fast as you can and after eight counts open the arms as wide as possible.

3. Repeat four times.

Watchpoints: Don't forget that back should be straight and stomach in.

Benefits: Excellent bust-firmer.

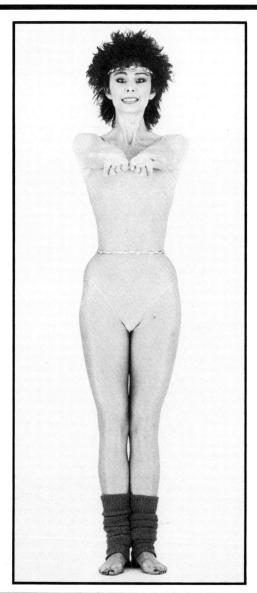
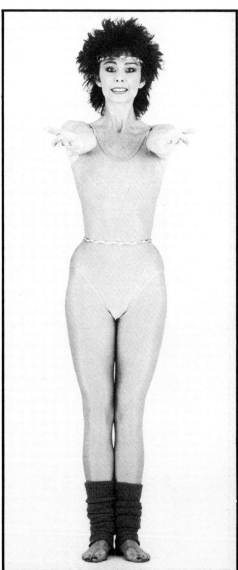

The KISS

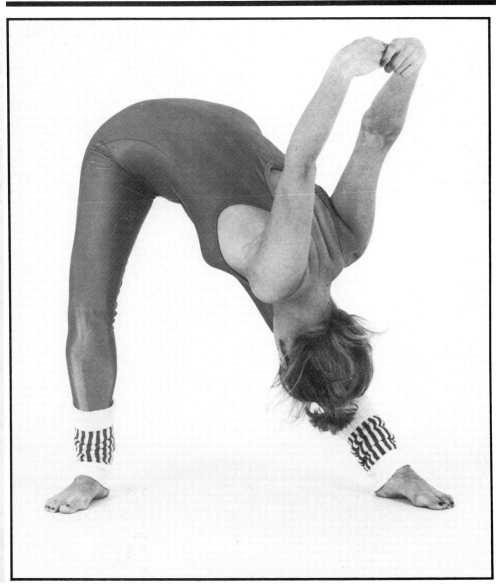

Starting position: Stand with legs apart and feet turned out. Clasp the hands behind the back.

Breathing: Breathe in as you stand straight, out as you reach forward.

1. Bend the left knee, keeping the hands clasped. Reach forward, try to get your head down on to your right knee and bring arms up behind you as far as you can. Bounce there three times, then back to starting position.

2. Repeat the movement, this time bending the right knee and getting your head down to touch your left knee. Bounce there three times then come back up.

3. Repeat 1 and 2, until you've done it eight times.

Watchpoints: Keep bent knee in line with foot.

Benefits: Loosens shoulders and hips, helping flexibility.

The **KISS**

EXERCISE FOUR (This exercise is not included on the KISS album)

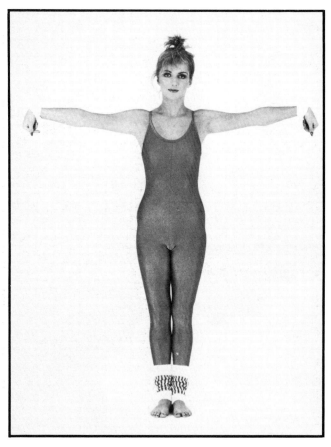 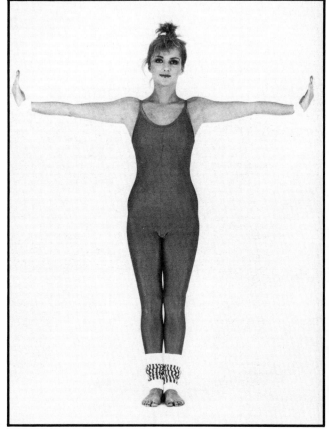

Starting position: Stand with the feet together and parallel. Make sure stomach is pulled in. Hold arms out to side at shoulder level, palms facing floor.

Breathing: Naturally throughout.

1. Curl your hands in trying to touch wrist with tips of fingers.

2. Uncurl hands by pushing fingertips high in the air and flexing the hands back.

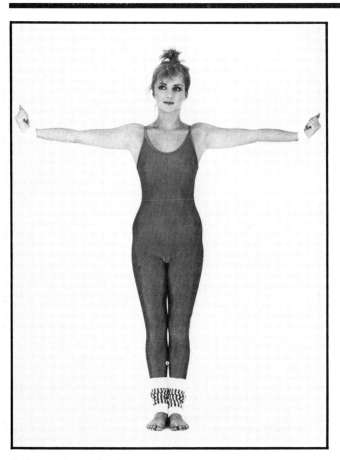

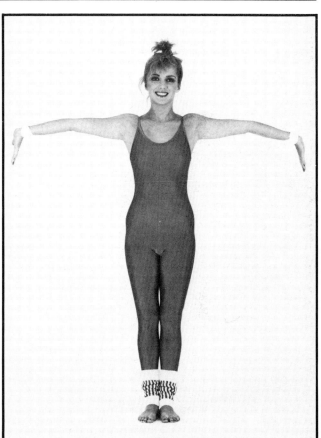

3. Repeat 1 and 2, eight times.

4. Turn palms to ceiling. Do the same curling, uncurling and flexing back eight times.

Watchpoints: For this exercise really to work, you've got to get further and further with each curl up and flex back, so push hard. Keep elbows really straight.

Benefits: Works the wrists, attacks flab on underarms, helps chest and shoulders.

The KISS

ON THE FLOOR— EXERCISE ONE

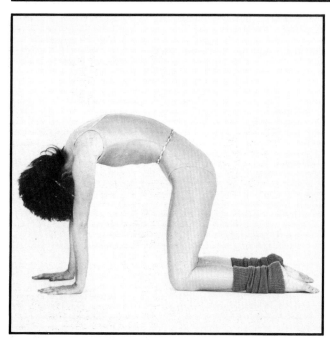 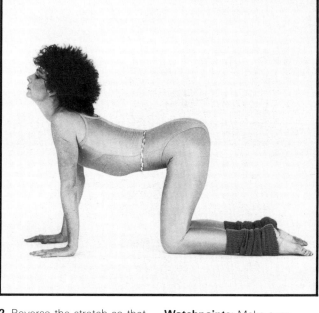

Starting position: Go down on all fours. Spine should be straight.

Breathing: Out as you round the back, and in as you arch down.

1. Round your back just like a cat would. Drop the head and pull in the stomach as if you were trying to get it to touch the spine.

2. Reverse the stretch so that your back is now hollowed and your head is high. Go back to first position and do the whole stretch four times solwly, then sixteen times fast.

Watchpoints: Make sure elbows are straight.

Benefits: Very good for the back.

EXERCISE TWO

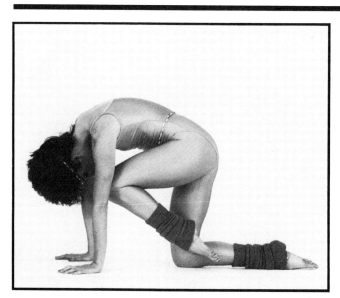

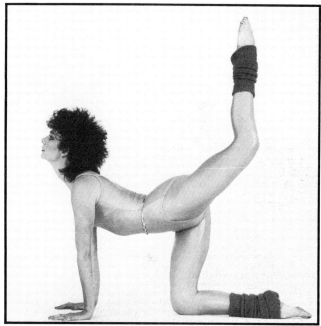

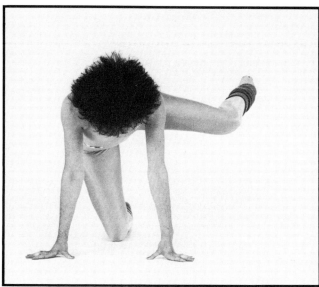

Starting position: Down on all fours with palms resting on the floor and spine straight.

Breathing: In as leg comes in, out as it extends.

1. Bring left knee in to touch the forehead, rounding the back and keeping elbows straight.

2. Extend left leg back and up, lifting head at same time. Go back to starting position. Do this eight times with each leg.

3. Lift your knee out to the side, keeping the knee bent. Lift to hip height. Do this sixteen times to each side.

Watchpoints: Don't sink sideways!

Benefits: Excellent for bottom, hips and waist.

The KISS

EXERCISE THREE

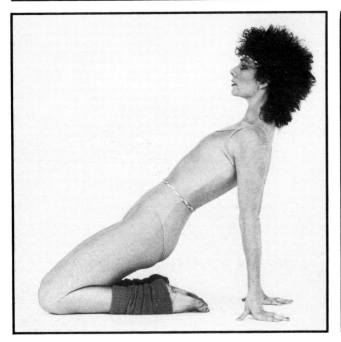 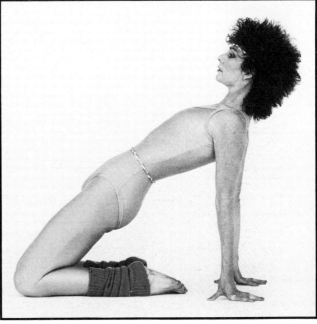

Starting position: Kneel with the knees slightly apart. Lean back and put your hands on the floor behind you.

Breathing: Steadily throughout.

1. Lift up with the thighs, so that bottom gets further away from your heels. Relax back. Do this sixteen times.

Watchpoint: Don't press up from the waist.

Benefits: Shapes and streamlines the thighs and tightens bottom.

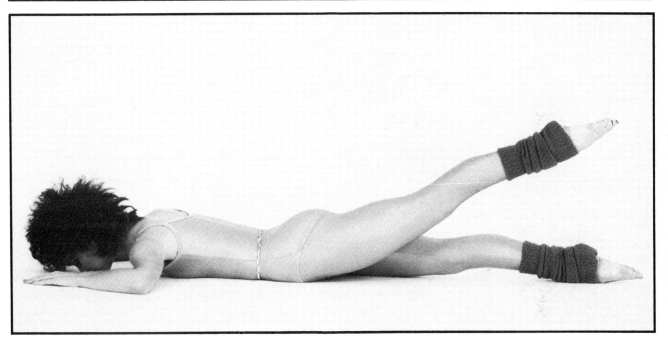

Starting position: Lie face down with feet together and toes pointed. Elbows should be bent and hands resting lightly on the floor level with your face.

Breathing: Out as you kick, in as you lower.

1. Kick right leg up sixteen times, making sure it stays behind you, then kick left leg up sixteen times. Keep your toes pointed all the way through.

Watchpoints: Keep the hips on the floor.

Benefits: This will strengthen the lower back and firm bottom.

The KISS

EXERCISE FIVE

Starting position: Lie on your stomach with legs stretched out and toes pointed. Arms are bent at elbows and hands resting easy on the floor at face level.

Breathing: In before you start, out as you scissor legs.

1. Raise your legs, keep hips on floor.

2. Open and close your legs like scissors, alternating right over left and left over right. Do sixteen of the scissor movements, then relax and repeat.

Watchpoints: Try to pull stomach off floor and keep hips down.

Benefits: Bottom, stomach and thighs.

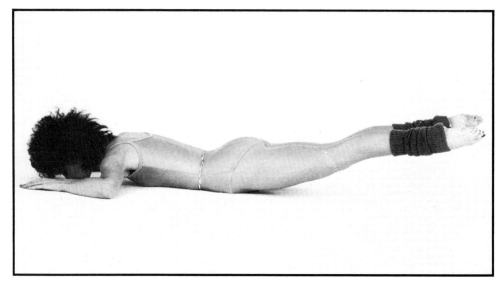

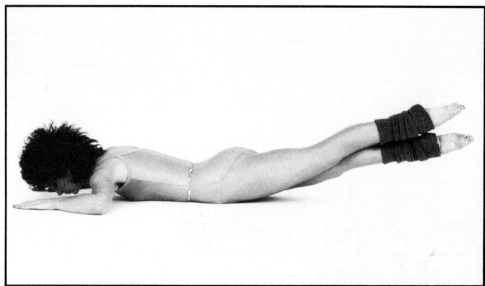

EXERCISE SIX

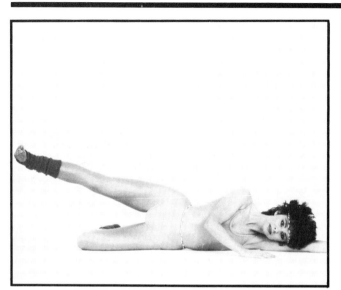

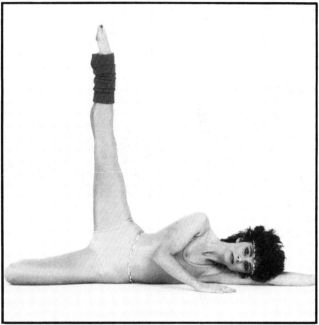

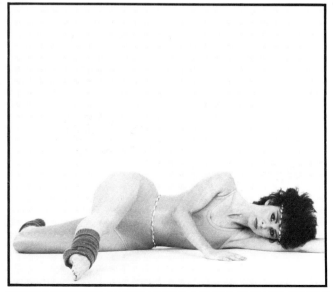

Starting position: Lie on your left side with the left leg bent and arms resting lightly on the floor.

Breathing: In as you raise leg; out as you lower it.

1. With foot flexed, raise your right leg up as high as you can, then back to start position. Do twenty-four raises.

2. Point toes and raise the leg; then bring it over and down to the ground in front of you. Raise leg up again. Do eight of these.

3. Roll over on to other side and repeat 1 and 2 all the way through.

Watchpoints: Make sure the knee doesn't bend as you raise your leg, and keep body straight and stomach in. This is a tough one!

Benefits: Inner and outer thighs.

The KISS

WORKOUT—EXERCISE ONE

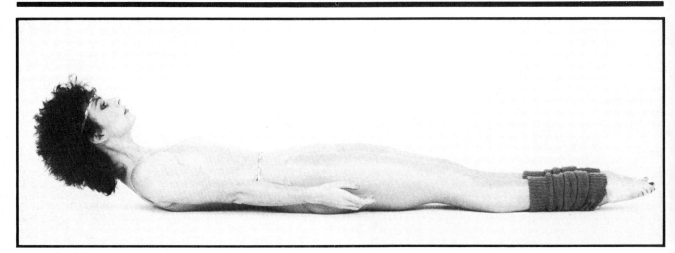

Starting position: Lie flat on your back with toes pointed and arms down by your sides. Make sure stomach is neatly tucked in and middle of the back is pressing down on to the floor.

Breathing: Out as leg is raised, in as leg is lowered.

1. Lift your head and shoulders off the ground so that you are looking straight ahead.

2. Do eight kicks up with the right leg, then eight kicks up with the left leg. Relax. Go back to starting position then repeat all the way through once more.

Watchpoints: Don't let your head drop back, and keep the neck relaxed.

Benefits: Flattens and firms the stomach.

Far Right:
Stylish, sexy, unmistakably 'Hot Gossip' – Arlene Phillips took some of her best students and formed the fabulous successful dance group.

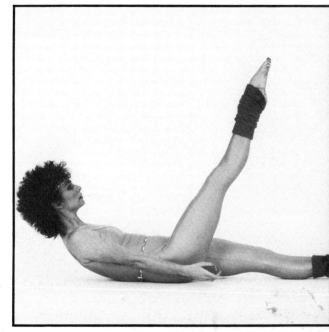

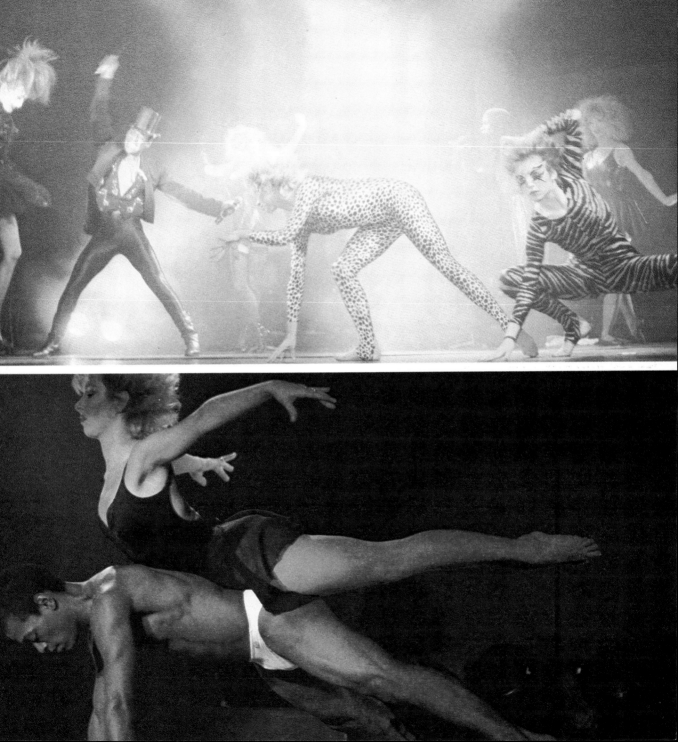

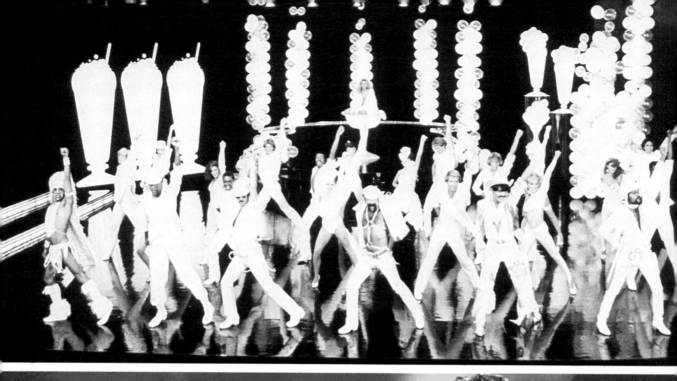
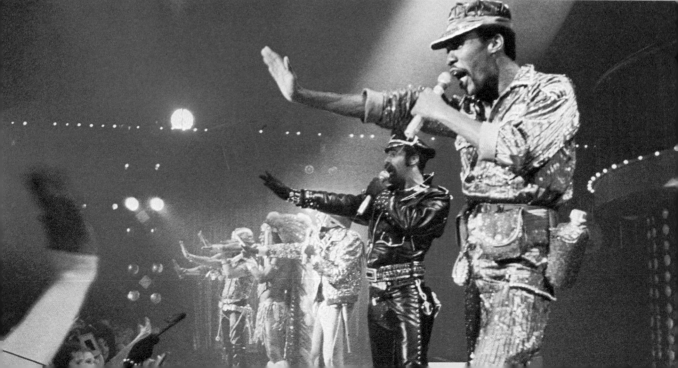

EXERCISE TWO

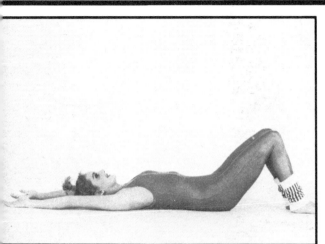

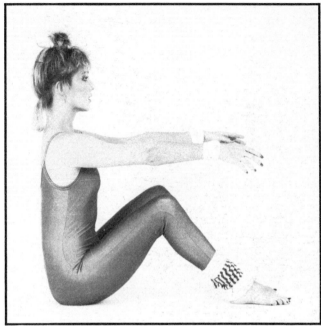

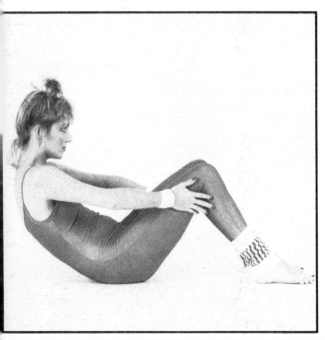

Starting position: Lie flat on your back with knees bent up and arms stretched out above your head.

Breathing: Out as you sit up, and in as you lower.

1. Start the slow sit-up bringing arms over the head and keeping the knees bent all the time.

Far Left:
The humour and style of 'Village People' made them great to work with. 'Can't Stop The Music' is the title of the film — I did stop when I took one week off during filming to have Alana.
(Thorn EMI Films Ltd)

2. Hold on to the thighs if you need to as you complete the roll up.

3. Slowly roll down to the floor again and back to starting position. Do the whole exercise sixteen times.

Watchpoints: This movement should be done slow and steady. Never crash back to the floor.

Benefits: A great workout for the upper abdominal muscles.

The KISS

EXERCISE THREE

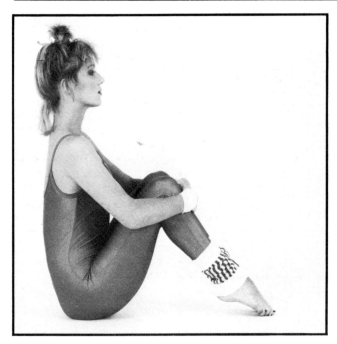
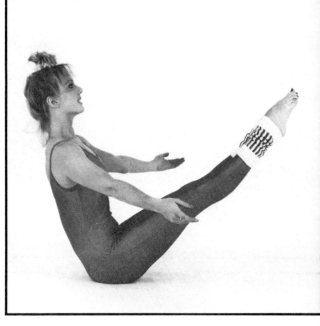

Starting position: Sit up, bringing hands round to hold thighs.

Breathing: Out as you extend legs, in as you lower.

1. Extend legs out to full stretch. Draw legs in again, trying to straighten spine at same time. Repeat sixteen times.

Watchpoints: If this hurts base of spine, rest on a folded towel.

Benefits: Stomach and legs.

EXERCISE FOUR

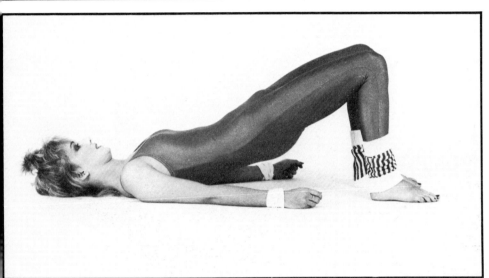

Starting position: Lie on your back with knees bent up, feet flat on the floor and hips' width apart. Let your arms relax by your sides.

Breathing: Out as you raise body and in as you lower.

1. Raise lower back off the floor and push with bottom to tuck under.

2. Come back to start position, repeat sixteen times. Relax, repeat another sixteen times.

Watchpoints: Try to isolate movement to hips and bottom. Don't push from the waist.

Benefits: Trims and firms bottom.

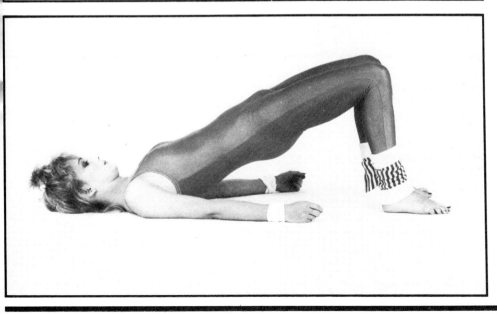

The KISS

EXERCISE FIVE

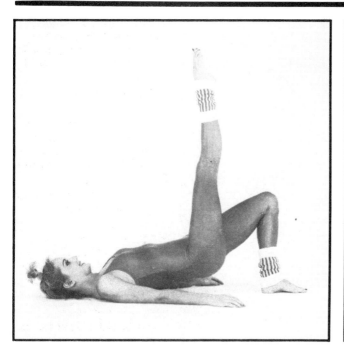 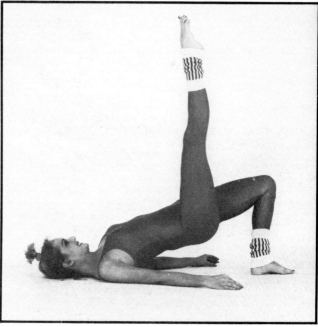

Starting position: Lie flat on back with arms by sides, knees bent, feet parallel and about hips' width apart.

Breathing: Out as you raise leg, and in as you lower.

1. Raise right leg, with toe pointed. Press hips up off the floor. Push under with your bottom as hard as you can, for a sixteen count, coming back to first position in between each count. Lower leg and relax.

2. Raise the left leg and lift bottom up off floor again. Keep pushing for a count of sixteen.

Watchpoints: Don't arch your back.

Benefits: Bottom and upper thighs get tight and trim.

EXERCISE SIX

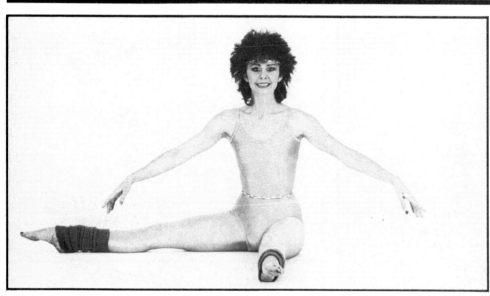

Starting position: Sit up straight with legs stretched out in front and toes pointed. Stomach and bottom should be pulled tight.

Breathing: Normally throughout.

1. Swing your right leg open as far as you can, keeping knees straight. Close together. Swing left leg open and close. Repeat.

2. Swing both legs open as far as you can. Close again, and repeat.

3. Repeat the whole exercise four times right through, getting legs more open each time.

Watchpoints: Make sure knees don't bend.

Benefits: Fights flab on inner thighs.

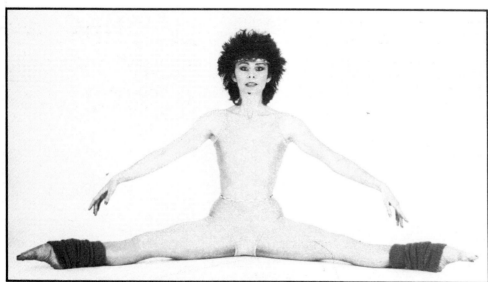

The KISS

EXERCISE SEVEN

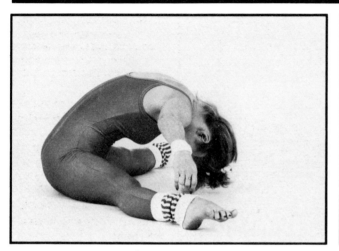

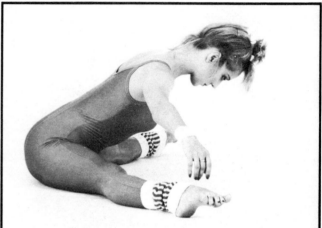

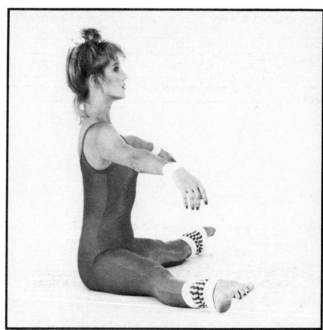

Starting position: Sit on the floor and open your legs as wide as you can; point the toes. Hold arms out at shoulder level.

Breathing: Out as you go down, in as you come up.

1. Round your back and roll down, trying to touch the floor with your head.

2. Stretch out spine as close to the floor as you can.

3. Sit up with a straight spine. Do all the way through four times.

Watchpoints: Keep head close to chest as you roll down; don't worry if you don't go very far at first—this one takes time!

Benefits: Waist and inner thighs get shapelier.

The KISS

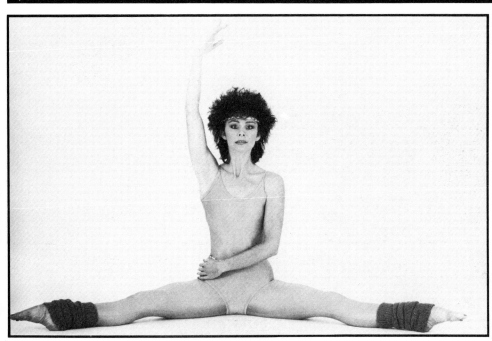

Starting position: Sitting on the floor with your legs as wide open as possible and toes pointed. Raise right arm above head. Left arm curves gently in front.

Breathing: In as you sit up, and out as you stretch over to the side.

1. Stretch over to the right leg, trying to get your ear close to your knee. Gently return to starting position.

2. Stretch over to the left leg.

3. Repeat all the way through eight times.

4. Relax forward as close to the floor as you can.

Watchpoints: Don't twist; go directly to the side.

Benefits: Wonderful for waist and inner thighs.

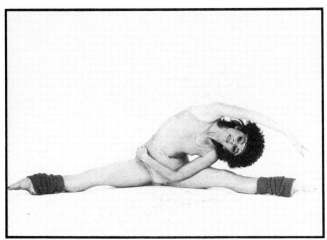

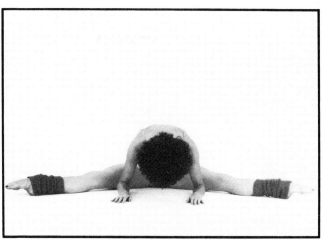

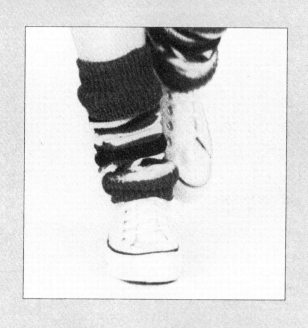

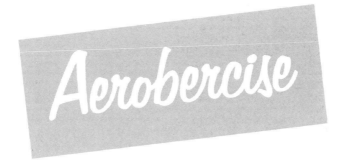

3

Aerobercise

AEROBERCISES

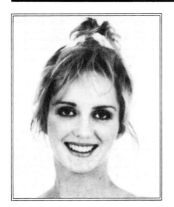

Jane Newman joins Bonita to take you through the KISS exercises. Jane is from 'Hot Gossip' – she was with the group for four exciting years – and is one of these people who is lovely to be with because she bubbles with enthusiasm and good humour. She thinks this is a welcome result of exercises and dancing which helps work off tensions and depression, and leaves you with a natural high. Jane is 29, her skin is in super condition, and she puts this down to the vitamin-rich eating plan that is all part of KISS.

Y ou've worked through KISS and now you're feeling supple, stretched…really good! It is time for the exercises which are designed to strengthen your heart and lungs by putting them into overdrive with non-stop action. The bonus from these aerobercises is that they raise the metabolic rate, helping you to burn up calories and burn off any surplus fat.

But before you even get into your running shoes—and, yes, it is essential to wear them for these exercises because your feet and ankles need good support—you *must* make sure you are really ready.

Any aerobic exercise is tough. Test your general fitness first. Go for a very brisk two mile walk. If you can't do that without feeling any strain, you are not ready for the aerobercises. Work hard on KISS and test yourself in another month's time.

Before you start check that your resting pulse is within the normal range. Make sure you're very relaxed when you do this. Rest the index and middle fingers of one hand on the inside wrist of the other, below the fleshy pad under the thumb. Don't use your thumb as it has a small pulse of its own and this can confuse the reading. Count the number of beats in 15 seconds, then multiply by four to find the number per minute. The average resting pulse comes in between 75 and 85 beats per minute. Higher than that and you're not ready for aerobercises. Lower than that is

Aerobercise

good—athletes often have a resting pulse as low as 50 beats per minute; this shows how efficient exercise has made their bodies.

The aim of aerobercises is to raise the pulse rate; but only to the level that is safe for you. Overdoing it could have fatal results. During the first four weeks of exercise, nobody should go beyond 125 beats per minute. And don't wait for the end of the session to do the testing, take your pulse after just one minute; this time count the beats for just 6 seconds, then multiply by ten. This is because the rate slows down so quickly when you stop moving. If it exceeds 125, stop. If you have high blood pressure and are taking medication, pulse readings will be distorted. Don't rely on them, and check with doctor about safe exercise levels.

After the first month you can raise your pulse rate gradually to:

AGE	MAXIMUM PULSE RATE DURING EXERCISE
20	160
25	155
30	150
35	147
40	145
45	140
50	135
55	130
60	125

The programme here will get you moving. When you can do it really easily, increase the time so you are on the move for twelve minutes. But don't go beyond that.

Work hard, but be realistic. You should get out of breath, but never so much that you can't hold a reasonable conversation (not too much puffing!) If you get really out of breath, the exercise isn't working as it should, because you can't get oxygen into your system. The results, far from being healthy, are dizziness and sickness, so stop.

After all these warnings, the good news! Aerobercises are going to be the most fun you've ever had during exercising.

Aerobercise

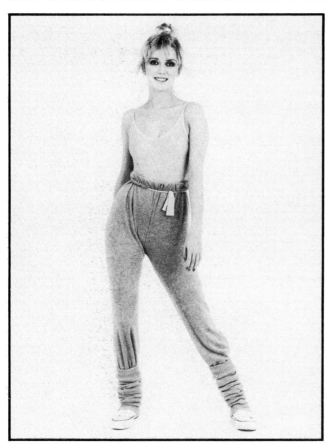

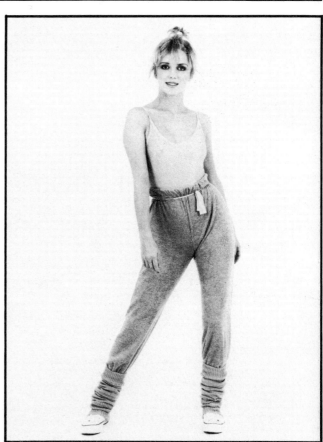

This is nonstop, right the way through, so keep moving and fill in any gaps with jogging. If it's your first time, don't forget the pulse test.

1. Stand with your feet apart and shift your weight from right to left, pushing hips from right to left at same time. Keep going. Thirty-two times very fast.

2. This time, as you move your hips, relax your head and neck from side to side. Sixteen times.

3. Now just the hips, but with two pushes each side. That's thirty-two double bumps.

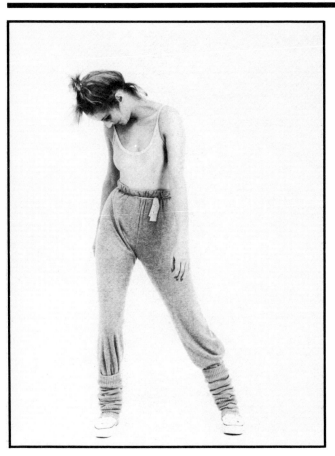

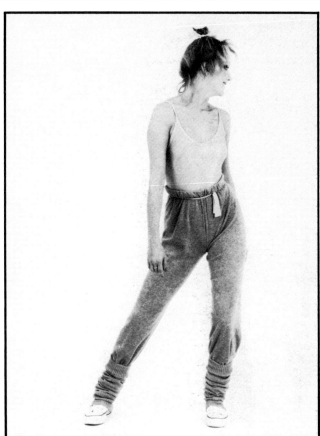

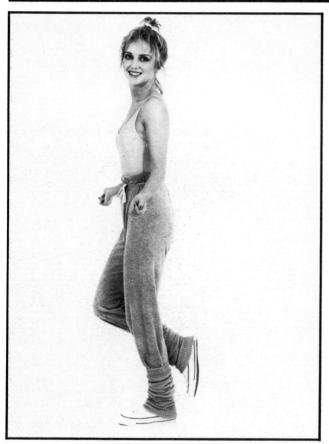

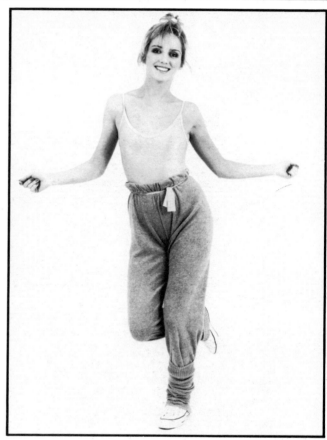

4. Now double bumps with the head movement as well. Sixteen times.

5. Pretend that you are holding a skipping rope and do a running skip. Don't forget to circle hard with the wrists. Thirty-two times.

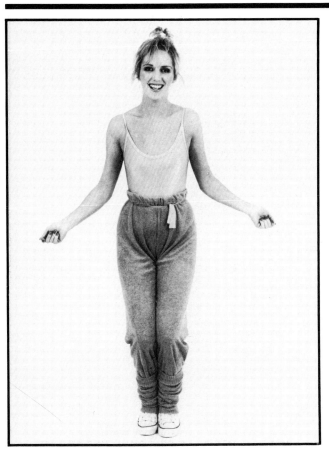

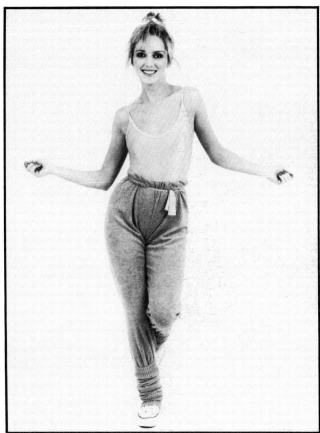

6. Now it's jumping rope with both feet together. Thirty-two times.

7. Go back to the running skip. This time pushing hips side to side. Thirty-two times.

Aerobercise

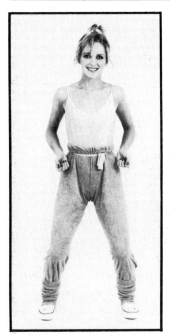

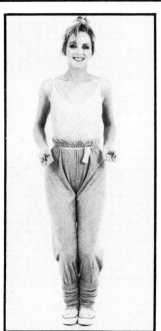

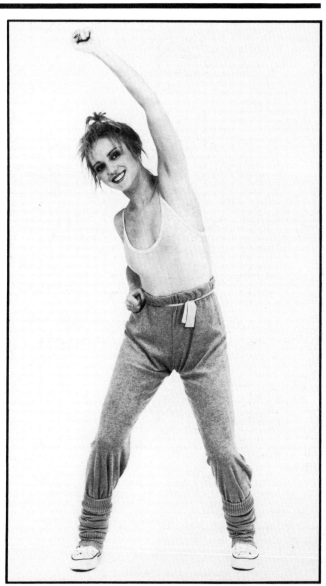

8. Jumping jacks: open and close your feet really wide. Sixteen times.

9. More jumping jacks and, as you open, punch your right arm up in the air and bring it down as you close; then the left. Sixteen times.

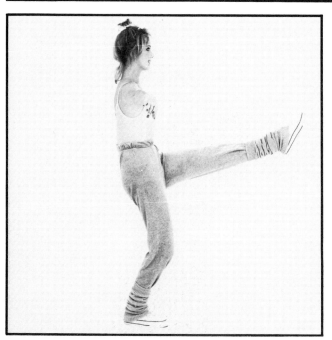

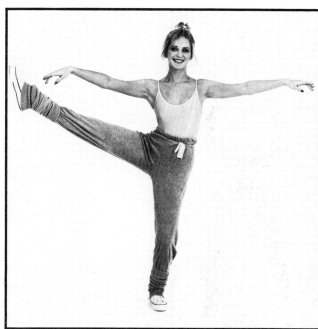

10. Small jump, both feet together. Jump on left leg and kick right leg to front. Repeat eight times. Then left eight times. Repeat, kicking leg to side, eight right, eight left. Then again to front, alternating right and left, sixteen times.

Aerobercise

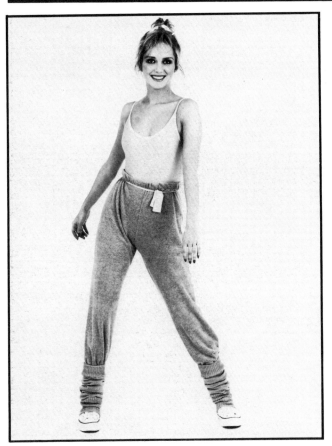

11. Step to the right. Jump and close the feet together. Step to the left, jump and close the feet together. Sixteen times.

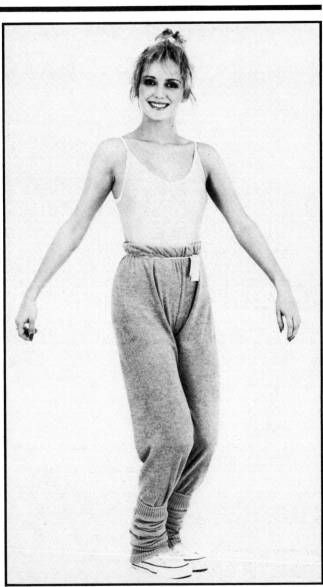

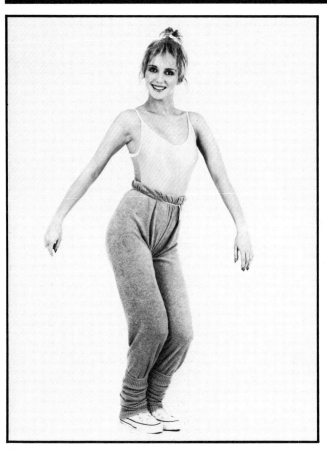

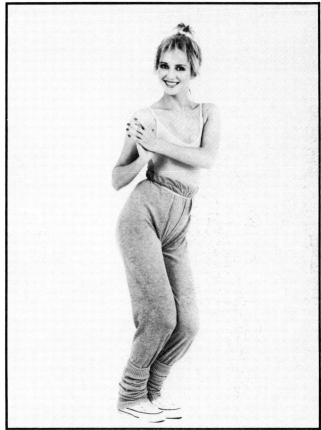

12. Repeat, pushing in to the hips as you land. Sixteen times. And then another sixteen times, this time clapping your hands as you land.

Remember: All the way through keep the rhythm, and fill in any pauses with jogging.

Progress: When you're really, really fit, you can go back to the beginning and work right the way through the sequence again, gradually increasing up to 12 minutes. That's the optimum time for the aerobercises.

Watchpoints: Make sure that as you land, you go through the ball of the foot to the heel, so that the foot is eventually flat. This means legs and feet are working as shock absorbers.

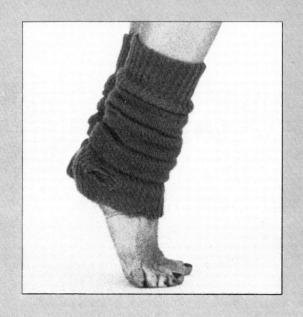

The Advanced KISS

THE ADVANCED KISS

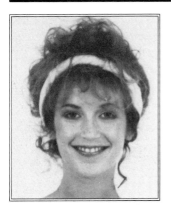

Kim Leeson takes you through The Advanced KISS. She trained with the Royal Ballet, but simply grew too shapely! Then she took classes with me at the Arts Educational School, and was so talented that I invited her to join 'Hot Gossip' four years ago. She is now 21 and our lead singer. Kim isn't naturally slim — but she works at it. She would never crash diet, which is why she likes my vitality diet. However late she gets home, she is scrupulous about cleansing off every scrap of make-up, then soap and lots of rinses with cool water before she puts on a light moisturiser.

One of the most rewarding aspects of teaching exercise and dance class for me is the way people improve. Even those who start out thinking they are hopeless can become star students! As a real challenge, this chapter contains some exercises which I have chosen because they are very tough.

When you get really good at KISS you'll be ready to have a try. With some people it will take three months, with others longer. But most people will get there in the end. And remember, the way to win the exercise game is to go at your *own* pace. The only competition is the challenges you set yourself. It is pointless fretting because someone you know can do the splits and you can't. You may not be able to do them today, but give them time...

The advanced KISS is not meant to replace KISS, but to supplement it and make it even more effective, to provide extra help to keep away that flab you've now got rid of.

Another of the bonuses of the complete KISS system is that it does great things for your skin and hair. You will work up a good sweat that will take wastes out of the body that otherwise could clog your pores. Exercise means more red cells in the blood and that means much better nourishment for the skin and hair. Exercise makes your skin supple too, and that means it's going to be more resistant to wrinkles and general sagging. Quite simply your skin is going to stay looking younger much longer.

Of course, it is wrong to exercise to the point where you are too exhausted to enjoy the rest of your life. But by now you've learned to listen to your body, so that is not going to happen, is it?

I will be finishing the exercise part of KISS by getting you moving the Hot Gossip way. This is where you *really* let yourself go, use all your new suppleness to move with the music. Don't forget to smile when you dance—this is the dancer's way to look twice as good.

When you have finished KISS it is important to cool down slowly; have a warm shower if you can, or wrap up in a tracksuit. If you cool down suddenly the muscles are more likely to get cramp or become sore. This is specially true if you've been sweating hard. Once you stop working your body, the sweat evaporates very quickly, leaving the skin cold, this cools the muscles very fast and the trouble can start.

After exercising, drink some water to replace what you've lost. At many dance centres they sell natural fruit juices. A glass after exercise tastes wonderful and it will replace the potassium and other minerals lost through sweating.

However many times a week you are doing your workout, don't think exercise is something you do and then finish. Try to get more movement into your life in general:

* Walk two miles every day (perhaps part of the way to work).
* Pretend that lifts and escalators haven't been invented.
* Don't sit for longer than 30 minutes in front of the television without getting up for a good stretch and a walk around. There is actually a condition called 'TV legs' where all that sitting in one position leads to a shortening of the hamstrings.

KISS cares about your body. Put you and KISS together and the results should be sensational!

The Advanced KISS

EXERCISE ONE

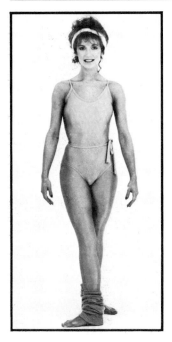

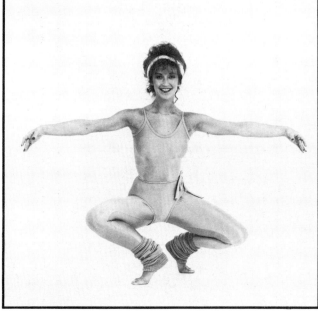

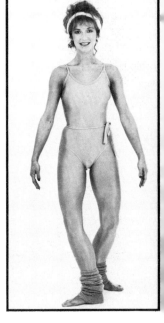

Starting position: Standing beautifully with arms held lightly by your sides, feet turned out and right leg in front of left.

Breathing: Out on the way down, and in on the way up.

1. Bend both knees, keeping heels on the floor all the time. Come up again and repeat.

2. Bend the knees again, this time go down low, letting both heels come slowly off the ground together. Have your weight distributed equally between right and left leg.

3. Do two more bends keeping your heels on the floor and then rise up on to the balls of your feet and hold for a count of eight. Lower.

4. Repeat all the way through twice.

5. Go through 1 to 4 again, but this time with the left leg in front of the right leg.

Watchpoints: Make sure you don't have weight on one leg.

Benefits: This one really works on the thighs. It's hard work, but you'll love the results.

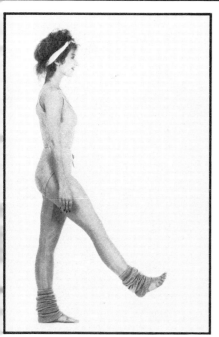

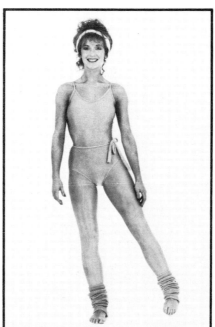

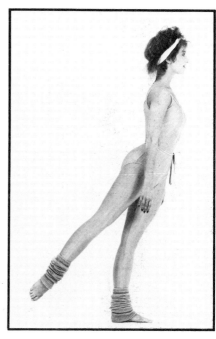

Starting position: Stand tall with arms naturally by your sides and right leg slightly raised.

Breathing: Naturally throughout.

1. Circle the ankle four times with the leg in front.

2. Circle the ankle four times with the leg held out at the side.

3. Circle the ankle four times with the leg at the back.

4. Change legs and repeat sequence.

5. All the way through twice more.

Watchpoints: Don't let the foot droop; make proper circles.

Benefits: Shapes ankles and calves.

The Advanced KISS

EXERCISE THREE

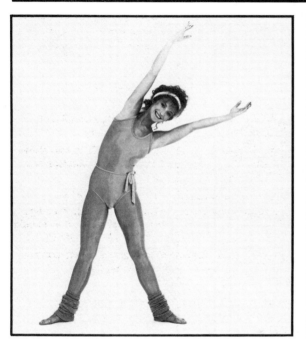

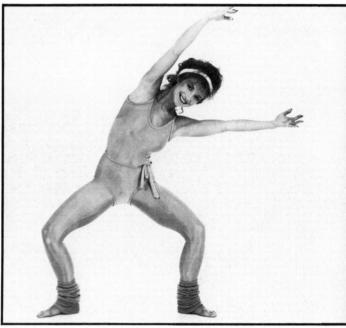

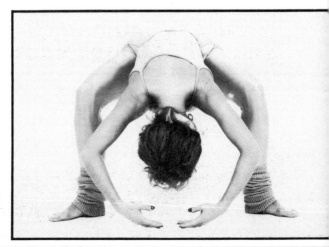

Starting position: Stand with the feet wide apart and pointed out. Arms by your sides. Check that stomach is pulled in.

Breathing: Out as you go down, in as you come up to the side.

1. Stretch to the left side of room with both arms, keeping both arms straight.

2. Drop the body forward down to the floor, relaxing knees as you go down really low.

3. Swing through and reach for the other side of the room.

4. Do the whole sequence eight times.

5. Go through the movement again; this time raise your right leg to the side as you reach for the left side of the room. Do this eight times through. Reverse it eight times.

Watchpoints: Stretch directly to the side; don't twist your body.

Benefits: Good for stomach, waist and thighs.

EXERCISE FOUR

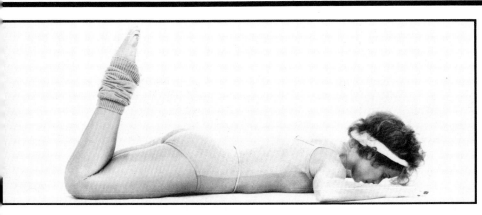

Starting position: Lie flat on your stomach with arms bent at the elbows and legs straight. Toes should be pointed.

Breathing: Normally throughout.

1. Bend knees and then lift thighs off the floor.

2. With the thighs still off the floor straighten the legs and very slowly lower.

3. Repeat eight times.

Watchpoints: Don't let legs crash to the floor, they should be lowered down slowly.

Benefits: Trims and tightens bottom and thighs.

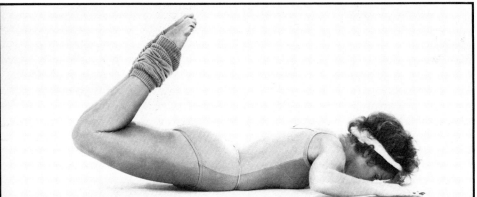

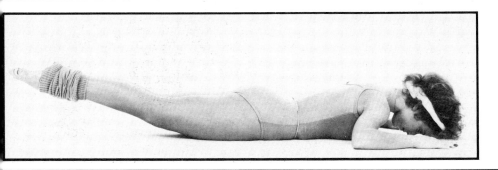

The Advanced KISS

EXERCISE FIVE

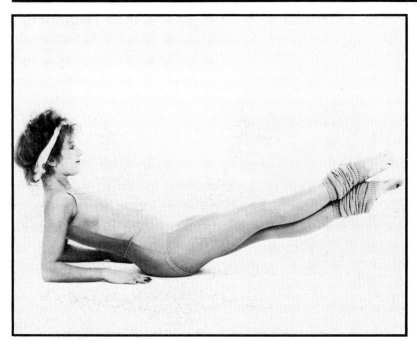 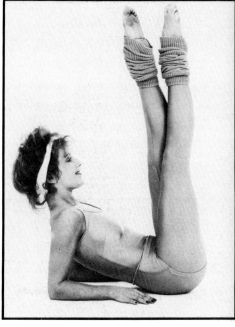

Starting position: Sit on the floor with both legs straight and knees facing ceiling. Lie back on your elbows. Support your lower back with your hands.

Breathing: Out as legs go up, and in as they come down again.

1. Make small scissor movements with your legs as you raise them up off the floor. Go up to a count of eight.

2. Lower the legs still making the small scissor movements for another count of eight.

3. Repeat four times, more when you build up your strength. Then try doing it without legs touching floor.

Watchpoints: Try to keep your body in a straight line and don't sag.

Benefits: Flattens stomach.

The Advanced KISS

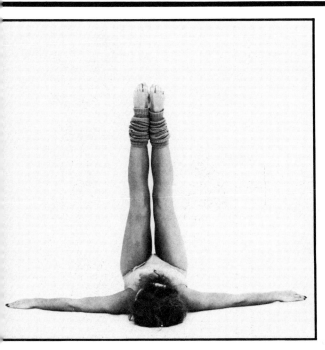

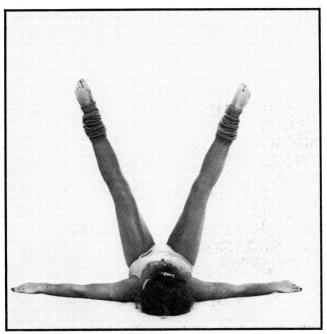

Starting position: Lie flat on your back with your arms extended out at the sides, legs stretched out, ankles together and toes pointed.

Breathing: Normally throughout.

1. Raise your legs at right angles to your body.

2. Open your legs, until you feel the pull, and close them again—aim for one hundred times when you get really strong.

Watchpoints: Make sure middle of back is flat on floor.

Benefits: Fantastic for inner and outer thighs and buttocks.

The Advanced KISS

AN ADVANCED KISS DANCE

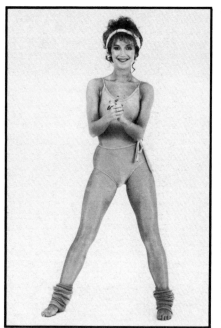 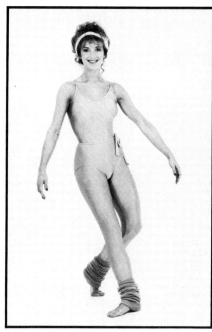 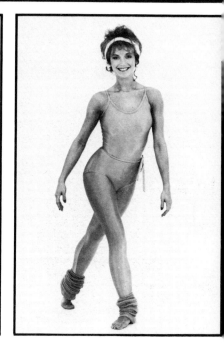

Starting position: Stand beautifully, with your arms naturally relaxed by your sides and feet together.

Breathing: Naturally throughout.

1. Step to the side really moving your hips.

2. Clap your hands.

3. Step back on the left leg on the ball of the foot.

4. Step forward on the right leg. Repeat to the other side. Then repeat sixteen times... So it's step on 1, clap on 2, step on 3, step on 4.

The Advanced KISS

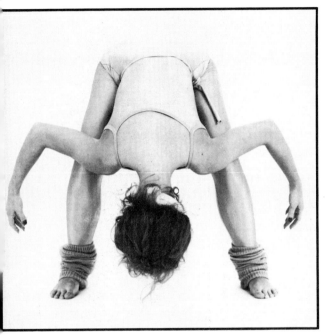 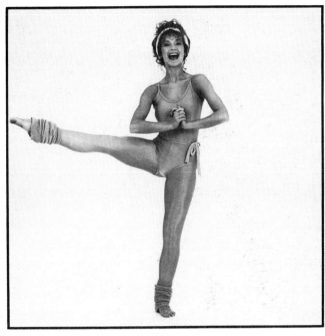

5. Repeat with a drop over on the count of 2 each time. So it's step on 1, drop on 2, step on 3, step on 4. Do this sixteen times.

6. Repeat 5 again with a kick as well as a clap on 2. So it's step on 1, kick and clap on 2, step on 3, step on 4. Do this sixteen times.

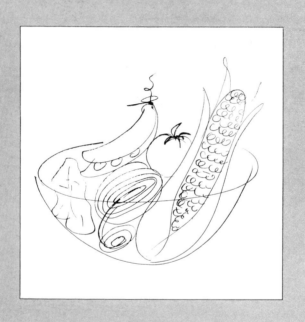

5

Diet for Life!

Diet for Life!

Do you hate dieting? From today you won't! This is day one of a 'super-food-plus' diet. You'll lose weight without ever feeling hungry, win a high-energy bonus and get the glow of good health that is the key to being beautiful. Best of all, once you've got slim, the plus-factor will *keep* you slim.

Ordinary diets might help you lose pounds of weight, but they don't help you make sure they stay lost. That is why out of every 100 women who diet, 96 soon regain the weight they've lost. Some start piling it back while they're still on an 'I'm starving diet'; others do as soon as they start eating normally. Don't worry; this won't happen with my 'super-food-plus' diet.

Simple calorie counting might help your arithmetic, but if it adds up to under 1000 calories a day your diet is doomed. As the latest American research shows, crash diets can in fact make your fat problems grow. Your body knows that its first job is to survive. Put it on starvation rations and it cleverly adapts. It puts a 'slow-down' on the rate at which it burns the calories. Its priority is to keep the fat reserves up in case of worse to come; this means you can stay just as fat although eating less.

The first strategy for getting out of the fat trap is to say 'no' to crash diets. The second strategy is to set a reasonable reduction in your calorie-intake. Eating 1200 calories for women, 1800 calories for men, are good starting points. Then add the plus factor from the 'super-food-plus' diet.

The plus factor is exercises that increase the speed with which you burn up those calories. When

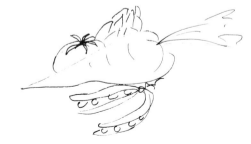

your body is stuck on slow-burn, you can, as I have said, get fat just by eating normally. It's simple equation: eat more than you burn and the extra is banked in your fat reserves. I have seen it happen to dancers I've worked with. They take a few months off, laze around, and the pounds pile on even though they're eating less than their normal work-diet.

Of course, real over-eating will make you fat. But doctors now believe those fatties who complain they eat no more than their slim sisters and still put on weight. True, they don't *eat* any more, but they *do* a lot less. Under-doing is just as vital a fat-factor as over-eating.

If you've been eating normally (check with my *Now you've got there, stay there later* in this chapter) why are you, say 7lb overweight? Every pound of excess fat equals 3,500 calories you haven't burned. To get that 7lb you have not used 24,500 calories. Taken over the year that is about 70 calories a day going into your fat-bank credit. If you're 10lb overweight that is around 100 calories a day going to fat. To calculate your fat-bank credit, just add a 0 to the pounts overweight you are.

Could you have used those calories? Yes! Just by doing the aerobercises in Chapter 3. They are not know as fat-burning exercises for nothing. Once you can do the whole 12-minute routine really well, you are burning 120 calories each time. And there is a bonus. After hard exercise, your body stays on the high-burn rate for a couple of hours after you have finished. Put more movement into your life and you will burn calories on the slim-person rate. That is the plus in the 'super-food-plus' diet. And the super-

food? It is just what it says. You are going to give your body the vitamin-rich, high-fibre, low fat fuel it thrives on with an eating plan that tastes terrific too. A diet for the getting the best out of life. This is why I have called this chapter Diet for Life!

Okay by now some of you will have your excuses ready so let's get *them* out of the way:

Diet for Life!

I can't get through a week of dieting without cheating; I've just got to pig-out. So it's no good me starting another diet because I won't stick to it.
Later in this chapter you'll find the 'diet-saver' to follow on the day after you have cheated on the diet. Stick with this binge-beater for just one day, then go back to the diet.

I'm doomed to be fat; my body just has too many fat cells.
Maybe, but it means you must work a little bit harder to reduce the amount of fat in them. And how did you count them? Very overweight people have been shown to have more fat cells, thought to come from overfeeding when they were babies (so don't be that cruel to your kids!).

I just don't have any brown fat to keep my weight normal.
Yes, the brown-fatters are lucky. The theory is that they take extra calories and, instead of converting them into fat, they turn them into heat. This means that however much they eat they don't get fat. You're not one of them, so turn up your fat-burner with my aerobercises and check the **How Hard Is Your Body Working?** chart at the end of this chapter. And you can forget about brown fat.

I haven't got time to exercise.
Exercise is a time-saver! Work out for half an hour and you'll then get through routine tasks twice as fast. And you can use your

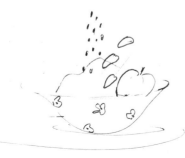

Diet for Life!

'work time' as exercise time. Walk part of the way to work every day, never use the lift, make up a dance routine to do with the vacuum cleaner (and never mind who gives you a funny look!). Do not slump in front of the TV, as I have said earlier, for more than 30 minutes at a time. Get up, have a good stretch, keep supple and keep burning those calories.

I dare not exercise because it will make me even hungrier.
Wrong; exercise produces chemical changes in the blood that will cut your appetite.

I don't mind eating less, but I am 45 and too old to exercise.
Exercise slows down the ageing process. Start gently with the Warm-Up (Chapter 1), stay with that for a month, then move on through the rest of the KISS programme. And exercise will pep up your mental alertness too.

I'm too tired to exercise as well as diet.
When I come home really tired, I do a 40-minute workout to restore my energy so that I can enjoy the evening. Exercise actually fights off tiredness. Other diets may have made you tired, but this one won't. It is vitamin and mineral-rich. Extra protection against fatigue is to step up potassium. Bananas are the best source; eat one a day when you're over-tired.

I am not really fat—it is just fluid retention.
Try drinking more water and taking in less salt—see the salt section in diet strategy later in this chapter.

Dieting just makes me depressed: I hate missing out!
The diet I recommend isn't a no-no. It's a positive thing you are doing for yourself to make you look good and feel great. Exercises are definitely mood-improvers.

Now we've got rid of all the excuses, let's get on and do it! First, find out how much you need to lose. The weight charts below are a good guide. But your best friend is a full-length mirror in front of which you can take the 'wobble test'.

Take off all your clothes (but women should keep on a good support bra). Stand in front of the mirror and jump up and down. Do it front and back. Did you see the fat actually wobbling? Check the backs of your arms, thighs, inside knees, and stomach for flab. If you look generally thin, but are still flabby, you don't need to cut calories. You need to go on to the Maximum Vitality Eating Plan (see later in this chapter) and concentrate on the shaping, firming exercises in the two KISS chapters (2 and 4).

Aim for a weight loss of around 2-3 lb a week. Don't just cut the calories. If you do, for every 3 lb you lose only 1 lb will be fat, the other 2 will be muscle tissue. You end up thinner, but saggy-looking. To end up slim and shapely, remember diet alone won't do it and exercise alone won't do it. But put the two of them together—wow!

Diet for Life!

WHAT HAVE YOU GOT TO LOSE?

Use these charts as a guide to what you should weigh. But remember, you're an individual, not an average, so 5lb either side could be perfect for you. If you cannot decide what frame you are choose the medium one. Heights are without shoes, and weights without clothes. Weigh yourself every morning before breakfast and remember that a weight swing of up to 5lb is normal. (Metric weights are given to their nearest whole number).

Women (over 18)

ft	in	(metres)	st	Small frame lb	(Kg)	st	Medium frame lb	(Kg)	st	Large frame lb	(Kg)
5	0	(1.52)	7	2	(45)	7	7	(47)	8	6	(53)
5	1	(1.55)	7	5	(46)	7	10	(49)	8	9	(54)
5	2	(1.57)	7	8	(48)	8	1	(51)	8	12	(56)
5	3	(1.60)	7	11	(50)	8	4	(52)	9	2	(58)
5	4	(1.63)	8	0	(51)	8	8	(54)	9	5	(59)
5	5	(1.65)	8	3	(52)	8	12	(56)	9	8	(61)
5	6	(1.68)	8	6	(53)	9	2	(58)	9	12	(62)
5	7	(1.70)	8	10	(55)	9	6	(60)	10	2	(64)
5	8	(1.73)	9	0	(57)	9	10	(61)	10	6	(66)
5	9	(1.75)	9	4	(59)	10	0	(63)	10	10	(68)
5	10	(1.78)	9	8	(61)	10	4	(65)	11	0	(69)
5	11	(1.80)	9	12	(62)	10	8	(67)	11	5	(72)
6	0	(1.83)	10	2	(64)	10	12	(69)	11	9	(74)

Diet for Life!

Men (over 18)

ft	in	(metres)	Small frame			Medium frame			Large frame		
			st	lb	(Kg)	st	lb	(Kg)	st	lb	(Kg)
5	3	(1.60)	8	5	(52)	9	2	(58)	10	0	(63)
5	4	(1.63)	8	8	(54)	9	5	(59)	10	4	(65)
5	5	(1.65)	8	11	(55)	9	8	(61)	10	6	(66)
5	6	(1.68)	9	0	(57)	10	0	(63)	10	11	(68)
5	7	(1.70)	9	4	(59)	10	3	(64)	11	2	(70)
5	8	(1.73)	9	8	(61)	10	6	(66)	11	7	(73)
5	9	(1.75)	10	0	(63)	10	10	(68)	11	12	(75)
5	10	(1.78)	10	4	(65)	11	0	(69)	12	2	(77)
5	11	(1.80)	10	8	(67)	11	4	(71)	12	6	(78)
6	0	(1.83)	11	0	(69)	11	8	(73)	12	11	(80)
6	1	(1.85)	11	4	(71)	12	0	(76)	13	1	(82)
6	2	(1.88)	11	8	(73)	12	3	(77)	13	6	(85)
6	3	(1.90)	11	11	(75)	12	8	(79)	13	10	(86)

Diet for Life!

THE SUPER-FOOD DIET
You'll gain health as you lose weight *recipe follows

	BREAKFAST	LUNCH (home or away)	DINNER
SUNDAY	Raw fruit muesli* with $\frac{1}{4}$ pint (150ml) skimmed milk	Wholemeal roll packed with 1 oz (25g) peanut butter and as much watercress as you like. $\frac{1}{4}$ pint (150ml) natural yogurt mixed with $\frac{1}{2}$oz (15g) chopped dates	Main meal pasta soup.* Half a charentais melon with 4oz (100g) raspberries
MONDAY	1 slice Bran health bread* with 2 sliced tomatoes and 2oz (50g) cottage cheese	2 slices wholemeal bread sandwiched with scraping low-fat spread, 2oz (50g) cooked and mashed butter beans, scraping of Marmite and lots of crisp lettuce. 1 apple	Brown rice and apricot pilaff* 4oz (100g) black grapes
TUESDAY	Raw fruit muesli* with $\frac{1}{4}$ pint (150ml) skimmed milk	Lunchbox salad: 3oz (75g) cooked red kidney beans, 1 small potato boiled in skin and diced, lots of lettuce, 1 tablespoon natural yogurt flavoured with 1 teaspoon tomato juice – as dressing. 1 orange	4oz (100g) grilled prawns with mustard on 2oz (50g) wholemeal pasta with orange and watercress salad. $\frac{1}{4}$ pint natural yogurt with $\frac{1}{2}$oz (15g) toasted almonds
WEDNESDAY	1 whole orange. 1 slice Bran health bread* topped with lightly-poached egg	Wholewheat pitta bread filled with 2oz (50g) hummus, raw cabbage and $\frac{1}{2}$oz (15g) unsalted peanuts. 1 banana	4oz (100g) grilled chicken livers with 3oz (75g) green grapes on 2oz (50g) cooked brown rice. Perfect baked apple*
THURSDAY	Raw fruit muesli* with $\frac{1}{4}$ pint (150ml) skimmed milk	Wholemeal roll filled with 1 ripe mashed banana mixed with $\frac{1}{2}$oz (15g) chopped dried figs and $\frac{1}{2}$oz (15g) finely crumbled walnuts. $\frac{1}{4}$ pint (150ml) natural yogurt	1 baked jacket potato with 2oz (50g) well-drained tuna fish and 1oz (25g) grated Edam cheese 4oz (100g) eating plums topped with 2 tablespoons natural yogurt
FRIDAY	$\frac{1}{2}$ grapefruit, grilled with bare teaspoon honey. 1 slice Bran health bread with 2oz (50g) cottage cheese, grilled	Italian Salad*. 1 chopped apple with $\frac{1}{2}$oz (15g) sultanas	Spinach and yogurt pie* 4oz crushed strawberries blended with $\frac{1}{4}$ pint (150ml) skimmed milk, $\frac{1}{2}$oz (15g) crushed almonds
SATURDAY	Raw fruit muesli* with $\frac{1}{4}$ pint (150ml) skimmed milk	2 slices wholemeal bread sandwiched with scraping of low-fat spread, 2oz (50g) cottage cheese, 1 chopped apple, 2 chopped sticks of celery, $\frac{1}{2}$oz (15g) chopped walnuts	Sesame fish kebabs* with 1 potato, boiled in its skin and 4oz (100g) barely-cooked whole French beans. $\frac{1}{2}$ small pineapple

Aim to lose between 2/3lb a week. If you are losing faster then increase the amount of food you are eating. This diet averages 1200 calories a day.
Insurance. Take 1 multi-vitamin pil and 1 multi-mineral pill every day.

RECIPES FOR SUCCESS

RAW FRUIT MUESLI
Preparation: 5 minutes
Serves one

---

1 tablespoon oat flakes

1 tablespoon bran

½oz (15g) almonds

½oz (15g) raisins

1 hard dessert apple

Put the oat flakes and bran in a cereal bowl. Grate the almonds into the bowl. Chop up the raisins and add them. Just before eating, core the apple (leave the peel on). Chop and add to the bowl. Remember as soon as you chop into a fruit, it starts to lose its food value, so always add the apple at the last moment.

BRAN HEALTH BREAD
Preparation: 25 minutes
(plus rising time)
Cooking time: 40 to 45 minutes
Makes 1 generous loaf

14oz (400g) wholemeal flour

1oz (25g) bran

1oz (25g) wheatgerm

1 level teaspoon fine sea salt

½oz (15g) fresh yeast

½ pint (300ml) warm water

1 tablespoon corn oil

1 dessertspoon molasses

Put the wholemeal flour in a large, warmed mixing bowl. Stir in the bran, wheatgerm and salt. Blend the yeast with the warm water and pour into the flour mixture. Add the oil and molasses and mix to make a dough. Adding bran can make the mixture a bit dry. You may need to add a little more warm water. If it's too sticky, add a touch more wholemeal flour.

Put the dough on a lightly-floured worktop and knead for 10 minutes. Slip the dough inside a large, lightly oiled polythene bag and leave in a warm place for 1 hour or until dough has doubled in size.

Knead the risen dough and shape into a round loaf. Put on a greased baking sheet. Cover and leave in a warm place until it has risen again.

When it looks nearly ready, turn on oven; set at 400°F (200°C) Gas 6. After 15 minutes, put bread in oven and cook for 40 to 45 minutes.

Transfer the cooked loaf to a wire rack and leave to cool.

This will be a close-textured loaf—full of flavour.

MAIN MEAL PASTA SOUP
Preparation: 10 minutes
Cooking: 20 to 25 minutes
Serves one

2oz (50g) fresh broad beans

1 small onion

1 large tomato

1 medium potato

¼ vegetable stock cube, dissolved in ¼ pint (150ml) boiling water

1 teaspoon fresh basil

Freshly-ground black pepper

1oz (25g) wholemeal pasta

Slices of fresh lemon

Shell the broad beans and put them in a saucepan. Skin and chop the onion, chop the tomato and potato (leave the skin on) and put them in the pan. Pour in the vegetable stock. Stir in the basil and a good shake of pepper. Simmer for 10 minutes then add the pasta and cook for another 10 to 15 minutes until the pasta is tender. Pour into a warmed soup bowl and float the slices of lemon on the top.

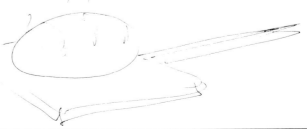

Diet for Life!

BROWN RICE AND APRICOT PILAFF
Preparation: 10 minutes
Cooking: 55 minutes
Serves one

½ small onion

½ small green pepper

2 teaspoons olive oil

2oz (50g) brown rice

¼ vegetable stock cube dissolved in ¼ pint (150ml) boiling water

1oz (25g) dried apricots

2oz (50g) smoked haddock

1oz (25g) Cheddar cheese

Skin and chop the onion; chop the green pepper. Heat the oil in a pan and fry the onion and green pepper for 4 minutes. Stir in the rice until it's thoroughly mixed with oil. Pour in the stock. Put a lid on the pan—it must be a good fit. Simmer for 20 minutes.

Chop up the apricots and mix with the rice in the pan. If the mixture is drying too quickly, add boiling water. Put lid on pan again and simmer for another 20 minutes, or until rice is tender and liquid is absorbed.

Flake the haddock and mix in. Heat through. Put on warm serving plate. Grate cheese over top and serve.

ITALIAN SALAD
Preparation: 10 minutes
Serves one

1oz (25g) wholewheat spaghetti rings, cooked and cooled

2oz (50g) sweetcorn, cooked and cooled

1 firm medium tomato

unlimited lettuce

2oz (50g) tender garden peas

1 tablespoon crunchy peanut butter

1 teaspoon fresh lemon juice

2 tablespoons boiling water

Put the spaghetti rings and sweetcorn in a bowl. Chop up the tomato and lettuce and add them with the peas.

Mix the peanut butter with the lemon juice and enough of the boiling water to make a sauce for the salad. Trickle it into the bowl—yummy!

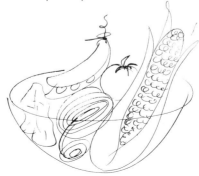

SPINACH AND YOGURT PIE
Preparation: 15 minutes
Cooking: 35 minutes
Serves one

1 good-sized potato

8oz (250g) fresh spinach

1 small tomato

2oz (50g) cottage cheese

2 tablespoons natural yogurt

Salt (if used)

Freshly ground black pepper

Don't peel the potato. Boil until almost (but not) tender. Cut into thin slices. Wash the spinach and cook in the water that clings to the leaves for 10 minutes. Drain as well as you can.

Preheat oven to 350°F (180°C) Gas 4. Use as little butter as possible to grease a small ovenproof dish.

Chop the tomato and mix it with the spinach, cottage cheese and yogurt. Add salt (if you use it) and pepper. Line the dish with half the potato slices. Add the spinach mixture then put rest of potato on top. Cook in the centre of the oven for 20 minutes then serve at once.

SESAME FISH KEBAB

Preparation: 10 minutes
(plus soaking time)
Cooking: 5 minutes
Serves one

1 tablespoon lemon juice
Salt (if used)
Freshly ground black pepper
1 teaspoon fresh chopped herbs
4oz (100g) cod
1 dessertspoon toasted sesame seeds

Preheat grill. Put lemon juice, salt (if used) and pepper in a small bowl. Stir in the herbs. Cut fish into chunks. Soak cod in the lemon mixture for 10 minutes.

Drain the cod and thread onto a skewer. Grill the fish for 5 minutes, turning the skewer as it cooks.

Coat with the toasted sesame seeds.

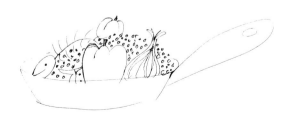

PERFECT BAKED APPLE

Preparation: 5 minutes
Cooking time: 40 minutes
Serves one

1 large cooking apple
½oz (15g) fine wholemeal breadcrumbs
¼oz (8g) dates
1 teaspoon honey
2 teaspoons hot water
Pinch of cinnamon

Preheat oven to 400°F (200°C) Gas 6. Core the apple and put it in an ovenproof dish. Put the breadcrumbs in a small bowl. Chop up the dates and mix with the breadcrumbs, honey, hot water and cinnamon. Spoon this into the core-hole of the apple.

Make a cut in the skin all the way round the fattest part of the apple. Cook in the preheated oven for 40 minutes or until very soft.

DIET-SAVER

Yesterday was awful, you pigged-out on chocolate and cheesecake. So today you are going on this cleansing diet so that tomorrow you can get back to the superfood diet—right!

Preparation: 5 minutes
Makes 1 day's supply

1 pint (550ml) tomato juice
1 raw egg
¼ pint (150ml) natural yogurt
1 teaspoon fresh chopped mint
½ teaspoon Marmite
1 pint (550ml) mineral water, like Evian
8oz (250g) green grapes

Blend the tomato juice with the egg, yogurt mint, Marmite and mineral water. Divide into four. Drink morning, lunchtime, early evening and late evening. Use grapes each time as a chaser.

Diet for Life!

MAXIMUM VITALITY EATING PLAN

This is your new way of eating. First when you lose weight with the 'super-food-plus' diet' (later in this chapter). Then for your happy, healthy, slim new life.

GET FRESH

You should eat fresh fruit and fresh vegetables every day. When skins are edible, eat them. Those vital vitamins and minerals are concentrated just under the skin — peel a potato and you are throwing the goodness away. The worst thing you can do to a vegetable is to overcook it, all the goodness will escape out into the water and end up down the sink. Eat vegetables raw when you can or cook them in the minimum amount of water.

Prepare raw fruit and vegetables just before eating. I've known people cut their breakfast grapefruit in half the night before. That means by morning over half the vitamin C has gone missing.

Fresh fruit and vegetables should make up the highest proportion of your diet — up to 60 per cent of what you eat.

GET FIBRE

Your fresh fruit and vegetables are rich in fibre. Now add more of that healthy, slimmer's friend with good amounts of wholefoods like wholemeal bread, oats, bran, brown rice, wholemeal pasta, peas, beans and lentils, jacket potatoes, nuts and dried fruits.

A few enlightened doctors, had been saying it for years, but it took the run-away success of Audrey Eyton's book *The F-Plan* to convince people that dietary fibre was good for you and could help you to lose weight.

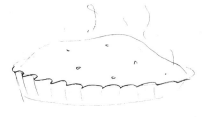

Diet for Life!

It seems a bit odd at first, that something you can't even digest is good for you — but fibre is. It doesn't give you any nutrients but its bulk (what used to be called roughage) is a vital part of the whole digestive process. It helps food to pass through the gut, protecting against the 'over-refined' diet problem: constipation. It's also thought to protect against cancers and diabetes.

In fact, it makes natural good sense to eat your foods 'whole' — as near to their natural condition as possible — with all the fibre left in. Though you won't digest the fibre, it will help you digest the nutrients in the food. This is because you have to chew more to get the high-fibre food down. A good chew means more saliva and gastric juices are produced to carry out the work of digesting the nutrients.

Fibre richly deserves its place in any healthy eating plan and it does slimmers plenty of favours. In fact, it's so filling that it's very difficult to over-eat. Low-fibre food just slips down, all too easily — compare a plate of high-fibre crunchy raw vegetables with a dish of ice cream. High-fibre makes sure you never feel hungry on the super-food diet.

PICK YOUR PROTEIN

Lean time for slimmers when it comes to meat — choose chicken and leave the skin, that's where the fat is. White fish is good and you get an excellent mix of proteins from cheese, eggs, skimmed milk, wholegrains, beans and nuts. Yogurt is part of every good eating plan. I eat it every day for protein and calcium — and it keep's intestinal flora in good condition — important for health and digestion.

TAKE CARE WITH FAT

Don't cut it out all together — you need it for the fat-soluble vitamins A, D and E. But remember fat makes fat. I keep it to a healthy minimum, getting what I need from eggs, cheese and nuts. I'm save on fat by using skimmed milk and low-fat spread on bread (or the barest scraping of butter).

DON'T PASS THE SALT

I never add salt to food, you can get what you need without doing that. If you're hooked on the flavour, try using the substitute called Ruthmol. Why no salt? British people eat far too much, more than 30 times their need. Too much salt in the body has been linked with high blood pressures and strokes. You might not reach for the salt so eagerly if you stop and think that salt can hold up to 35 times its own weight in water. And who wants to be bloated?

SUGAR: YOUR FALSE FRIEND

Yes, it does give you a surge of energy, but then it takes away more than it gives you. It uses up your own stocks of vitamins and minerals and leaves you tired, even irritable. It has no place in my healthy-eating plan. Use honey instead.

WATER WELL

Drink eight glasses a day. It's essential to your inner health and the good looks of your skin. If you don't like tap water, try sparkling Perrier water or Evian. Still not hooked? Add a slice of orange. Drinking just before you eat will help stop you feeling hungry. I never drink more than two cups of coffee a day — caffeine is another false friend that gives you just a temporary life. Persevere with herb teas, or try the grain coffee-substitutes.

Diet for Life!

NOW YOU'VE GOT THERE, STAY THERE

You've dieted and exercised down to your perfect weight. Now stay there by adding to the super-food diet — working out your own calorie needs. Keep with the exercises and increase your food intake. Weight for weight, men need more calories: less of their body weight is fat and so they use more calories to keep warm. To find your total, multiply your weight (in pounds) by 16 for a woman, 17.5 for a man, to get your daily allowance. Not got your calculator handy? Here's a guide. If you want to eat more, then exercise more (see next chart).

weight			Calories	Calories
st	lb	(kg)	for women	for men
7	0	(44)	1568	1715
7	7	(47)	1680	1837
8	0	(51)	1792	1960
8	7	(53)	1904	2082
9	0	(57)	2016	2205
9	7	(59)	2128	2327
10	0	(63)	2240	2450
10	7	(66)	2352	2572
11	0	(69)	2464	2695
11	7	(72)	2576	2817
12	0	(75)	2688	2940
12	7	(79)		3062
13	0	(82)		3185
13	7	(85)		3307
14	0	(88)		3430

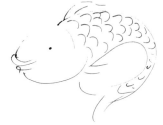

Diet for Life!

HOW HARD IS YOUR BODY WORKING?

When you're fast asleep, your body is still at work, building, repairing, breathing, digesting — using an average 1 calorie per minute. You get up and your calorie rate goes up. For most people, keeping all the bodily processes ticking over uses around 1500 calories a day. Your activity rate is added on to that. Balance calorie input (how much you eat) with calorie output (how much energy you burn) for stable weight.

Calories used in one minute

Under 5	6 to 7	8 to 10
cooking	bicycling	Arlene's aerobercises
driving	tough gardening	energetic sex
golf	hard housework	jazz dancing
knitting	jogging	running
typing	horse-riding	skipping
walking slow	tennis	squash
washing-up	walking fast	swimming, fast

FIT FOR LIFE

Staying with the basic strategy of the maximum vitality eating plan, you can now start planning your own personalised super-diet. Expand on the ideas in the super-food diet and if you want more help — have a look at two of my own top favourite cook books. *The Here's Health Cookbook* by Carol Hunter (Heinemann) and *The High-Fibre Cookbook* by Pamela Westland (Martin Dunitz).

Remember that a good diet for health is a balancing act that gives you everything you need every day. You should have protein every day — normal portions of lean meat or fish and make sure you include liver once a week. Other good sources are eggs (but not more than four a week) nuts and pulses. For calcium, A D vitamins, and useful protein, include milk products — especially yogurt. The best and brightest way to the B vitamins and the carbohydrates you need the wholegrain foods. Most of all, be really generous with fruit and vegetables for those vital vitamins and minerals. Don't forget that means every day for leafy green vegetables, citrus fruits and a good selection of other vegetables and fruits. The more you mix it — the better!

Remember the wrong foods make you weak and weary. The right foods, the maximum vitality foods, will make you feel good and look terrific: fit for life!

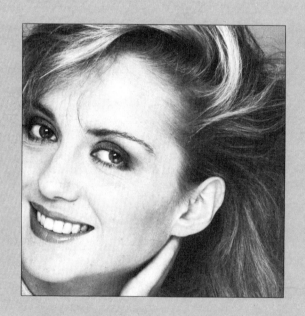

Right:
What I insist on when I'm working is attack
– that means hard graft until it's perfect.
These star students do just that: Leo Sayer,
Wayne Sleep, Olivia Newton-John, Lulu,
David Essex and Pamela Stephenson.

I was very excited when the Americans
chose me to choreograph and do the
musical staging for 'Annie'. Highlights were
teaching Albert Finney to tap dance and
working with the children. (Columbia Pictures)

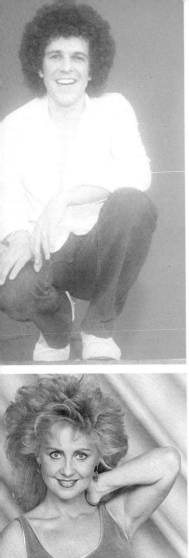
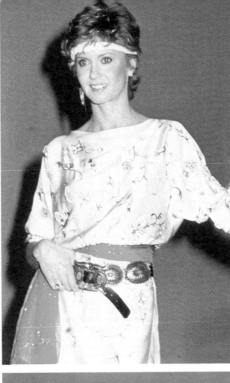
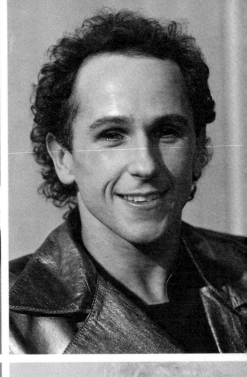
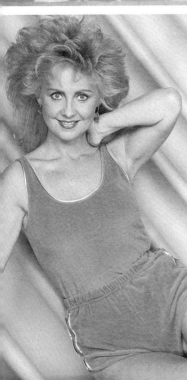
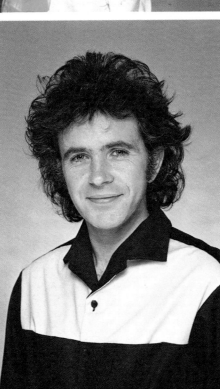
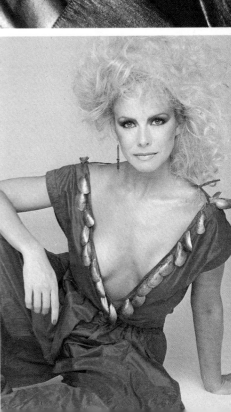

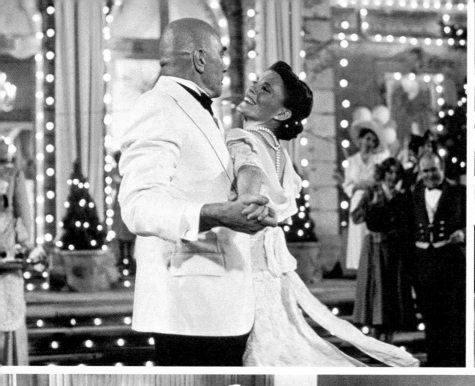
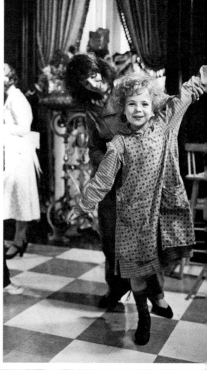
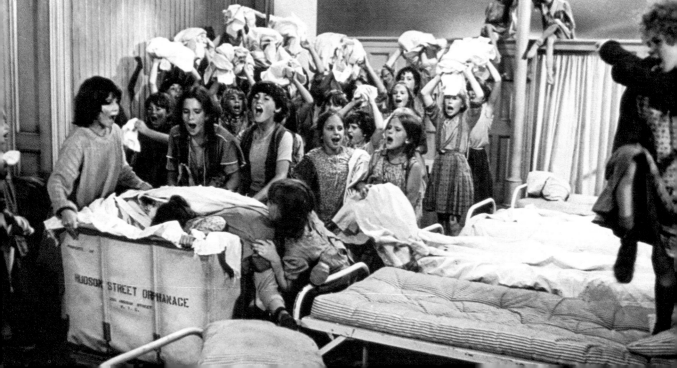

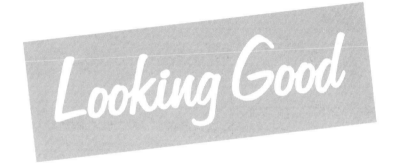

6

Looking Good

Looking Good

When people start taking classes with me they often gain something they're not expecting: a dramatic improvement in their skin condition. The cells in the skin need nourishment from the blood. If you don't exercise, only the minimum of blood reaches the skin; most of it meanders around in the central part of the body. Exercise gets the blood moving, and much more of it powers its way to the skin. Exercise increases the number of red blood cells, which carry oxygen to the tissues. Quite simply, when you exercise, your circulation is working at maximum efficiency. The skin gets more nutrients, and it looks better, and has a younger texture and tone.

Exercise warms the skin from the inside. This stimulates the production of collagen and elastin, the materials of the inner layer of skin, responsible for its strength and elasticity. The newest research in Russia and America shows that people with a regular, high level of exercise develop stronger, thicker and more supple skins—and that means skin much more resistant to wrinkles!

The muscle-stretching exercises in KISS will stimulate the skin, and help it to become thicker. The aerobercises (Chapter 3) will really get your circulation going, bringing the maximum nourishment to your skin. This is the first line of attack in order to get your skin in its best possible condition. The face and neck exercises in this chapter provide extra

Looking Good

help for specific areas.

Genes determine what sort of skin you are born with, its texture, its colour, and where it is programmed to wrinkle. But what happens to your skin is your responsibility. You can have young-looking skin at 40, or elderly, dingy-skin at 25—it is up to you!

I put exercise top of my skin-saver list. But exercise needs to be backed up with a good knowledge of your skin's major enemies, the importance of a good diet, plus daily cleansing and nourishing routines. These make up the formula for 'saving' your face, and it works. Here are some of the skin-spoilers.

Smoking. If you smoke you probably get very bored by people telling you to give up, so I won't! You know the health risks. But did you know that smokers wrinkle more rapidly? Lines around the mouth are deepened by drawing in the smoke, and habitual squinting round the eyes to avoid the smoke helps create your crows feet. More insidiously, the carbon monoxide reduces the amount of oxygen in your red blood cells, the ones that are responsible for getting the nutrients to your skin. So every time you light up, you put your skin on starvation rations. That means it ages more rapidly. Smoking is also thought to destroy collagen.

Sunning. Always use a water-resistant sun cream on your body and a high-factor sun screen on your face. A suntan you get through sunburn may fade, but the damage does not. Sunlight can damage skin cells so they no longer renew themselves. Damaged cells come to the surface of the skin, they harden and thicken, and the skin looks like crumpled leather. The right amount of sun with the right amount of protection can make you look terrific. Too much sun damages your skin for good. Skin looks ancient, and skin cancers may develop. All the rules that apply to the sun also apply to sunlamps.

Inadequate sleep. It is when you are asleep that skin renews itself most quickly. Find the amount of sleep your body naturally needs (anything from five hours to nine hours), and stay with it. During sleep the muscles are relaxed and skin rests on a smooth 'bed', it is not stretched and strained. Simply lifting your head to look at the ceiling can stretch the skin of the throat more than two inches; it needs sleeptime to recover.

Rapid weight loss. If you lose more than 3lb a week, the skin cannot shrink fast enough to fit your new shape. You may be slimmer, but you will also be saggy.

Too great a weight loss. A layer of fat naturally supports the skin; lose too much of this and your skin will fit your body like a loose, wrinkled stocking.

Central heating and air-conditioning. They create an unnaturally dry atmosphere which steals most of the moisture from the skin, which then becomes dry and tough—the first

Looking Good

step to wrinkles. A humidifier, or even a bowl of water on your desk, is a skin-saver.

The good news about skin is that its recovery rate is excellent. It responds to good treatment almost immediately. Now for a strategy for superb skin...

Water is its first need. Drink at least six glasses a day. If you find the taste of tap water boring, try one of the bottled waters. If it seems like a chore, buy yourself a beautiful glass to drink out of!

Check your diet. Vitamin C is vital; are you having really fresh citrus fruit and green vegetables every day? Have you switched to wholegrain bread for its B and E vitamins? Are you getting protein from lean meats, fish and eggs?

Skin needs to be thoroughly cleaned on a daily basis. Surface dirt and stale make-up left on the skin will soon make even the best of skins look dingy. I clean my greasy skin with Quickies Cleansing Pads, but liquid-cleanser and rinse-off cleansing bars work just as well. Skin toners should always be gentle, even with greasy skin. If you try to remove every trace of natural grease your skin (programmed to be greasy) will only work overtime to get more protective grease on to its surface.

Dry skins should stay with a cream cleanser. If you must wash with soap, remember that although soap doesn't harm your skin, not rinsing it off properly does and can lead to flakiness.

Daily cleaning needs to be boosted by a once-a-week 'rough' treatment to get rid of the dead cells on the surface of the skin which give it a dull look and conceal the fresh skin underneath. This is easiest to see in black women where it shows up as a sort of dusty grey layer. But whatever your shade, it is there and it has to go! It needs some kind of abrasive; a loofah will do it, or a Buf Puff. If your skin isn't used to this treatment, go easy at first. Use the loofah on your face for just one minute.

About once a month is right for a steam clean to open up the pores and let the debris float out that would otherwise turn into blackheads. Fill a bowl with boiling water and sprinkle some camomile into it. Hold your face over the bowl (but not too close or you'll be poached!) and make a tent with a towel. Stay there for three minutes. Let your skin rest for 5 minutes, then use a face pack designated for your skin type.

Do moisturizers lie? Only in the name, as there is no way of putting moisture back into the skin. If moisture could get into the skin, think how your hands would swell up every time you put them in water. But moisturizers are vital; they stop the moisture getting out of the skin. A healthy skin is about 90% water and it is the water-content that makes it smooth and softly-plump. Moisturizers work rather like the cling wrapping on a piece of Cheddar cheese which keeps it moist and fresh-looking in the fridge. Think how quickly the cheese gets dried up without its wrapping and you'll see why all skin needs moisturizer. Yes, even greasy skins. It's the lightest of liquids for them, going through to the rich creams for dry skin.

You'll get the most from your moisturizer if you apply it to slightly damp skin. The second job of any moisturizer is to keep out all the pollutants in the air.

What brand should you use? The only rule is, one you have heard of. This rule applies to cosmetics, too. Remember those imported eye-shadows no-one had heard of, that turned out to contain lead? It seems to suit my face to switch brands every so often. At present I'm using Estée Lauder prescriptives to care for my skin, but I know I can get good results from the much cheaper brands, too. Perhaps I'm just rather susceptible to pretty packaging!

Of course, skin care doesn't stop at the face. The next one down—your neck—is even more vital! Think about the skin of your legs: it has nice big muscles to lie on, but the neck skin is not so well-supported. It has to rely on a series of puny muscles and tendons. And think how much that skin gets stretched. It should be included in all your face-care routines. Remember the skin here is drier than your face and can age at double the speed. Help it to get the most from nourishing creams by massaging them in, always working from collarbone to jaw.

What part of your body is older than you are? Answer: elbows. When you bend them the skin is dramatically stretched; when you lean on them it is under pressure—it can age three times faster than the rest of you. A once-a-week soak in hot oil is an excellent therapy. Elbows should also be included in your daily hand-cream routine.

Hands contain very little natural oil and should be fed every day. Over-hot water and harsh detergents will strip the oil out of them, permanently, so avoid it. Your hand-cream routine is easier to remember if you keep a tube by the sink.

Rear admirable? Bottoms weren't really designed to sit on. The pressure of your body weight, plus clothes rubbing against them often causes the skin to get permanent goose pimples. Keep the fabrics next to them natural (silk or cotton) and don't wear tight trousers too often. This inhibits circulation and encourages dimpling. Fight this with a stern massage with a loofah, always in the direction of the heart. Don't forget to soothe generously with body lotion afterwards. This is the after-bathing treat for the whole of your body. And never spend too long in the bath—about 15 minutes is the limit. Soaking too long in water dries up the skin.

Could your thighs be nicer? Whether the dimpled-fat that sticks on thighs is cellulite (though some doctors claim it doesn't exist) or just fat, it doesn't help your skin look good.

Looking Good

Sea-salt on a rough-textured bath mitt, rubbed in vigorously (always towards the heart), can help smooth it.

Could beauty care be a complete waste of time? It could be, if you're not doing the very best for your teeth. The teeth are vital to the muscle tone and shape of the face. Without teeth, the chin gets nearer the nose and deep lines develop. The lip-line collapses. Most dentists believe that with proper care most people could keep their teeth, and it is the care you give your teeth every day that really counts. It takes only 24 hours for plaque to get its destructive hold. You should spend at least 10 minutes a day on your teeth; if you do not, you are bidding them a slow goodbye. When you brush your teeth, don't put too much toothpaste on the brush at once, it will make you want to spit and rinse too soon—you will think you have finished cleaning your teeth. The toothpaste should be used on a dry brush; wetting it makes the bristles less effective. Make sure your brush makes full contact with every surface and curve of each tooth and you'll be making a good job of it. Brush two or three teeth at a time, giving each section at least 10 strokes. Ask your dentist to show you how to use floss and an interspace brush; techniques vary from mouth to mouth. Sweet and sour are enemies of teeth. Sugar leads to the destruction of teeth and too much acid (drinking lemon juice or eating too many grapefruit) erodes the enamel on the teeth.

Homecare should be backed up with six-monthly check-ups—to me that's the most important beauty-date in my diary.

Who needs make-up? From what I have seen, most women look better with it. The strong look I use on-stage for Hot Gossip often breaks the make-up rules. It's designed to look startling but I'm not suggesting that it is an everyday look!

I'm always surprised when I see women shopping for make-up—whilst wearing it. I always go bare-faced to buy foundation so I can try it on my face, which is, after all, where I am going to wear it. I take a mirror with me and look at the effect under the artificial shoplights, and in the natural light outside. Greasy skins (like mine) are best with a matt foundation. Liquid foundations suit most skins in their 20s and 30s. Dry skins like cream make-up (it's another chance to moisturize). A good rule is the older you are, the lighter in texture the foundation should be and the lighter the coating of powder should be.

A lot of beauty books describe how you should reshape your face to get it as near as possible to oval. If you must, the rule is simple, darken an area and it will appear to recede, lighten it and it will be more prominent. But I think if your face is square, let it stay square. Complement the healthy glow that exercise (you have started haven't you?) and a good diet have put back in your cheeks with blusher. Look yourself right in the eye and start the blush directly below the centre of each eyeball taking it upwards to the temples stopping short of the hairline.

Bloodshot eyes are not beautiful, however much eye make-up you use. Smoky rooms and too much alcohol could be the cause. If they are persistently red and sore, check with your doctor. Are you screwing up your eyes so you can read this page more easily? You are helping create crows feet—get your eyes tested properly. You should exercise your eyes, especially if you are doing a lot of reading. Every hour or so, spend just a few seconds looking to each side, then up and down. Put your hands over your eyes for one minute and think black... Doesn't that feel better?

Eyeshadows—not really for eyes? Matching the colour of your eyeshadow to your eyes rarely works. It has to look good with your face. The only way to be sure is to put it on, stand back and have a good look. There just are not any rules about who should wear what. Buy small sizes, in cream, powder and pencil, and find out which you handle best. I don't believe in trying to change the shape of the eyes too much. But small tricks are effective: lining the rim of the lower lid with a white pencil to make eyes look bigger is good, and lifting droopy eyes with a triangle of colour on the outer half of the lid. You'll find your shadow-shaping by experiment. A good starting shape is to put the colour all over the top lid and about halfway along the lower lid. Smudge the colour up to the brow bone. Need more definition? Line the upper lid, then smudge it; use a kohl pencil on the inner rim of the lower lid. Several coats of mascara are better than one thick one that can look like fat spiders.

When your lips change colour... They do it with the weather, and with your menstrual cycle, so you can't expect even your favourite lipstick to look right all the time. Again, the lipstick has to look good against your skin and not match the colour of your lips. Breaking the rules with unnatural lip colour can be extra effective—black lipstick can be fantastic (but probably not on the bus first thing in the morning!)

SKIN	LIPSTICK
Fair skin	*all shades* of peach, rust and pink *lighter* reds and burgundies
Medium	*all shades* of rust, red and burgundy *lighter* brown and plum *darker* pink
Dark	*all shades* of red *lighter* bronze and plum *darker* red and pink

Looking Good

Mouth to mouth: make sure foundation covers lips; this will help lipstick stay where it belongs. Get a good outline with a pencil or a brush, then apply colour with a brush. Daytime gloss should be on the lower lip, otherwise you will look as if you have been eating a bag of chips in the dark while you were wearing boxing gloves.

Help yourself to healthy hair! Exercise is going to help by getting the nutrients from the bloodstream into the follicles in the scalp. Each hair on your head grows from its own follicle; its growth rate is about half an inch every four weeks; every day about 100 hairs fall out, and they need replacing. That is a heavy workload, and nutrition (to fuel the work) is obviously vital. Hair, like skin, is made of a protein called keratin and needs oil and moisture to stay healthy. Each hair is made up of three layers. The outer layer is called the cuticle; it is made up of tiny overlapping scales. Shiny hair means the scales are lying straight and reflecting the light. Mistreatment can disrupt the tiny scales; they are no longer flat and smooth and the hair no longer shines.

Are the following a regular part of your diet? Wholemeal bread, lean meat, fish and seafood, yogurt, liver, fresh fruit and vegetables? If the answer is yes and you are exercising and if your hair is still dull, try taking up to six brewer's yeast tablets a day to step up your B vitamins. And take a multi-mineral tablet every day (check the label and make sure it contains zinc).

Any of these can spoil the condition of your hair: alcohol, too much tea and coffee, and stress (see the next chapter for stress-fighters). All of these steal the B vitamins that should be going to help your hair. Smoking destroys vitamin C and this is also vital for hair health.

It sounds a bit odd, but if you spend five minutes a day standing on your head it will help your hair by improving blood flow to the scalp. It should help un-tense the scalp. But if it feels tight, you may need to do a regular scalp massage once a week. Use your fingertips in circular motions, keeping contact all the time with the scalp until you feel it move easily. Then move on to the next section until the whole of the scalp is relaxed and warm. Work with your head dropped forward and start at the nape of the neck.

My hair certainly does not have an easy life. I make up for that by giving it the best possible care. Once a month I give it a deep, conditioning treat with almond oil or Vitamin E oil before shampooing. Yes, it is messy—but it works! The oil should be just warm and is massaged into the ends of the hair and the scalp. Cover it with a plastic cap and leave for an hour, or longer. The best way to wash it out is to add a little shampoo and work that in before, gradually, adding the water. A few more rinses than usual and my hair feels revitalized and is very shiny.

Of course I do not use the same shampoo and

conditioner every time. Like everyone else my hair—and its needs—change with the weather, with hormone levels, with how hard I am pushing myself at work. Today's shampoos are so clearly labelled that it is easy to find what you need. I keep a good selection in my bathroom so I can give my hair exactly what it needs when it needs it. When work commitments mean I am washing my hair every day, I choose a gentle shampoo, either one marked for frequent use or a baby shampoo. Other times I use a shampoo specially for colour-treated hair. As well as the once-a-month oil treatment, I use a conditioner after each wash, but I just apply it to the ends of my hair.

How you shampoo matters. Gently brush first of all to get the oil and debris loosened from the scalp (but never brush wet hair, it can stretch it so much that it breaks). Don't use too much shampoo, and always apply with the hands, and not from the bottle. No rough rubbing; just gentle massage movements. Rinse very thoroughly with warm (never hot) water before conditioning. It is a waste of time to put conditioner on hair that's still full of shampoo.

Check that you've rinsed off the conditioner properly by looking at your hair—it should be shining when it's wet. Comb wet hair very gently and use the minimum amount of heat to dry it.

POSITIVE ACTION FOR GREASY HAIR

1. Use a mild shampoo and concentrate on washing the hair and not the scalp. Very hot water will encourage oil flow, as will shampoos that are very harsh.
2. Go easy on brushing the hair, and when you do your scalp massage, dip your fingertips in a solution of four tablespoons of luke-warm water and one tablespoon of fresh lemon juice.
3. Blow dry on warm setting. Hot air stimulates oil flow.
4. Avoid dry shampoos; they make greasy hair worse.
5. A light perm or colouring will tend to dry the hair—just what you need!

POSITIVE ACTION FOR DRY HAIR

1. Use one application of a mild shampoo and follow with a rich conditioner.
2. Once a week massage with warm olive oil (about two tablespoons) and leave the oil on for thirty minutes before shampooing it off.
3. Use a hair-dryer and heated rollers as rarely as possible.
4. Dry hair is often fragile—so brush and comb with respect. Never use a brush with hard bristles; check it on the back of your hand.
5. Whilst your hair is suffering from dryness, don't go for permanent colour tints or perms; the chemicals penetrate to the inner layer of hair and some moisture is lost. Get your hair in good condition first.

POSITIVE ACTION FOR NORMAL HAIR

1. Wash and condition your hair when it needs it (anything from every day to once a week).
2. Be reasonable with hair-dryers and heated rollers.
3. Your hair will take colouring, but don't overprocess it.

Looking Good

If you are not sure about colouring your hair, start with a shampoo-in colour that is not a permanent change. Do remember that the colour on the packet cannot be a totally accurate guide to what you get, you cannot know what colour the model's hair was before the colour went on, and all hair takes colour differently. For your first go, choose a colour close to your own.

I like my colour to be a little wild—so you can guess I've been using spray-on crazy colour since it was first invented! But if you want a colour-change that will just make you look better, think about your eye and hair colour. If you have the darkest olive skin and very black eyes, you are going to look strange with light blonde hair (but if that's how you want to look, fine). If strange isn't how you want to look, start your experiments just a few shades away from your natural colour. Most hair colourists agree that very dark colours accentuate lines on your face, and they don't flatter skin that has grown paler or more sallow (as skin tends to when it turns 30). Going a shade lighter usually flatters.

The best product advice here, as with cosmetics, is always buy a brand you have heard of and study the labels and instructions, which are there to help you.

HAIR COLOURING—HOW FAR DO YOU WANT TO GO?

Type	Effect	Life
Temporary rinses. Water soluble dye; does not penetrate the hair shaft	Adds warmth and depth and highlights natural colour	Until next wash
Crazy colour sprays. Metallic fragments of colour stick on the hair	Most dramatic effects on lighter shades of hair	Brushes or washes out, but may leave invisible traces for weeks that could affect application of other types of colour
Semi-permanent; penetrates the outer layer of the hair	Gives a darker and richer colour and can add shine. Test on small patch of skin to make sure you're not allergic	Up to 12 washes
Permanent tint; penetrates the inner layer of hair where it takes out pigmentation and adds new colour	Hair can be up to three shades lighter or darker. Do a patch test and follow packet instructions scrupulously	Re-growth means tinting at roots after four to six weeks
Highlights/lowlights; hydrogen peroxide or colour solution used on fine sections	Adds sunshine effect to light hair and subtle contrasting tones to darker hair	Roots will need retouching after three to four months

If condition is what you are working towards, then a blunt cut is going to help. This exposes the minimum amount of the ends of the hair, whilst cutting at an angle flares out the ends. And it is the ends that are most vulnerable to moisture loss and splitting.

You know your hair, so be realistic about what it can do. If, for instance, it's fine and thin, it can look miserable if you try to grow it really long. Instead, keep it around chin length and concentrate on condition, shine and cut. Work out how much time you are willing to spend on your hair. If you can only cope with a wash-and-wear style, tell your hairdresser. Your style is the business of you and your hairdresser, and no book can show it to you. It is a blend of what your hair will do, what shape your face is—and, more important than all that, your personality.

Because a lot of my life is spent teaching exercise classes (and that means working at least as hard as the students) or working with dancers when I'm choreographing, I like my hair long enough to tie out of the way when I want to. Sweatbands are essential if you're going to take your exercises very seriously, especially when you get on to the aerobercises.

I think of sweatbands as part of my live-in clothes. Of course, I have proper skirts that come to just the right length below the knee to wear when I'm visiting schools for my daughter. I have my wild clothes for parties and extravagant outfits for film premieres. But basic Arlene is really dance clothes—jogging suits, leotards, sweatshirts, and so on. I like the lively, energetic look and feel of them and they are also the healthiest clothes to wear.

You really should wear clothes you can move easily in. Tight clothes hamper circulation and make your muscles tense up. Imagine yourself buttoned into a coat that is far too tight across the shoulders and too cosy round your neck. Can't you feel the muscles at the back of your neck tense up in answer? And that is the first stage of a headache.

Tight jeans are terrific, but not for every day. They can cause the abdominal muscles to go into spasm and interfere with digestion. Stockings and tights that you can 'feel' are probably interfering with circulation, and that could lead to a crop of varicose veins.

Wearing tight clothes when you exercise is very unwise—and possibly dangerous. If you are starting out overweight and bulging you might not be ready to stand in front of a mirror looking at all that! So cover up with a tracksuit. Over the weeks and months as your new shape starts to emerge, start working out in footless tights and a tracksuit top. Then move on to a leotard—by now you will be looking great and feeling great, so watch yourself and enjoy yourself.

Looking Good

MAKE-UP—MAKING IT PERFECT

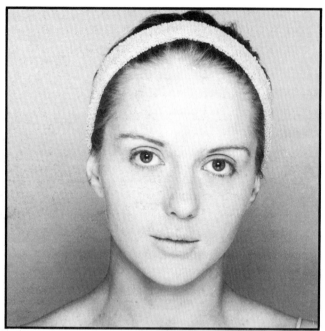

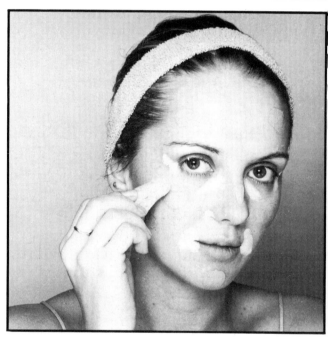

1. Start with completely clean skin and allow moisturizer five to seven minutes to be absorbed. If you don't use moisturizer, the foundation may be patchy, as thirsty skin absorbs the moisture from it. Spread foundation evenly, using the tips of your fingers.

2. Put concealer over dark shadows under the eyes and to minimize the smile lines around the mouth. Use a slightly damp sponge to blend concealer with the foundation. Remove any excess by blotting with a tissue.

3. Powder, and then remove excess with a very large, soft brush. Make sure it is soft so that foundation is not marked.

4. The effect of the eyeshadow is intensified by a soft pencil line along the upper lid and the inner rim of the lower lid. Be very gentle; never pull the delicate flesh around the eyes.

5. Blusher starts mid-way along the cheek, directly below the very centre of the eye. Take it right out to the temples for a healthy glow. Apply lipstick and just a little gloss. A light spray with Evian water will 'set' the make-up and help it to last.

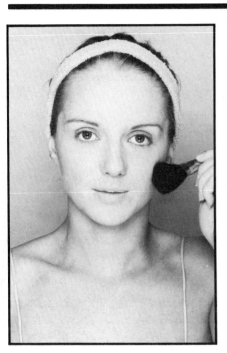

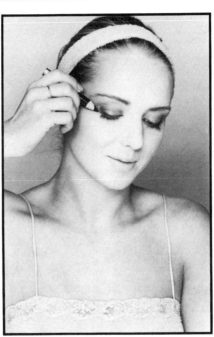

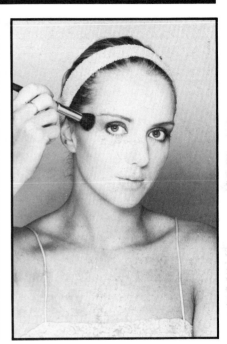

Looking Good

HAPPY HAIR

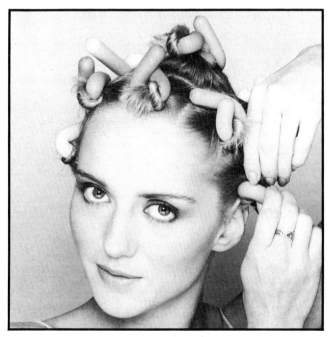

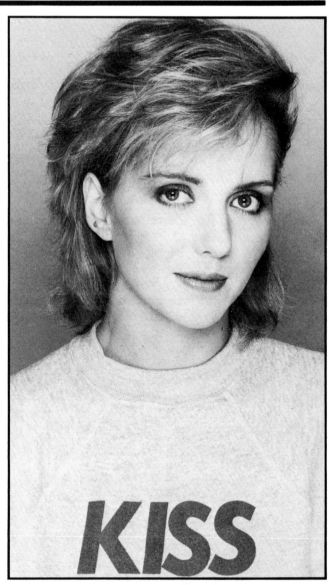

1. Jane is using Schumi Shapers to give her fine hair body and lift. These look like giant multi-coloured sausages, but they are wire covered with foam rubber. You can get a similar effect by wrapping lots of cotton wool round pipe cleaners. Jane sprayed her dry hair lightly with setting lotion and then took small sections of hair and twisted them before rolling them up on the shapers.

2. After 15 minutes, Jane took the shapers out; they made ringlet shaped curls. She smoothed her hair with her fingertips into a very natural looking style with lots of body.

MASSAGE

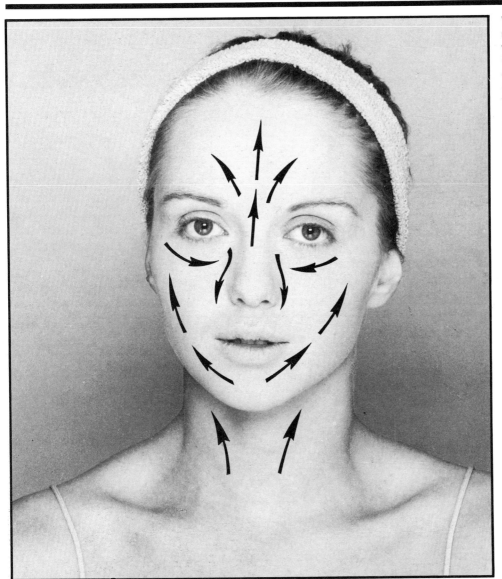

When you apply moisturizer or nightcream you can help it work extra well by massaging it in. Work with a slightly damp skin. Dot the cream all over your face; warm your fingertips and make small circular movements following the direction of the arrows and starting at throat level.

Looking Good

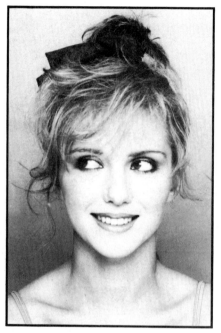 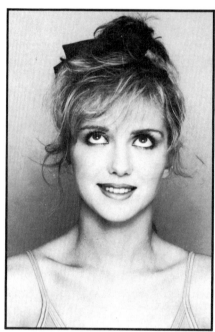 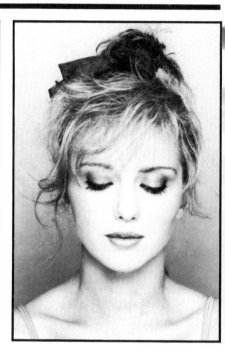

The Eyes Have It: Look right and left and up and down. It's an effective eye-refresher course. Do this for a few seconds every hour or so while you're working.

Right:
Kim Leeson is lead singer with 'Hot Gossip'.
She is showing how effective a single colour scheme can be. The subtle, yet strong, effect comes from using the same pink on cheeks, eyes and lips, truly sensational with her red-gold hair.

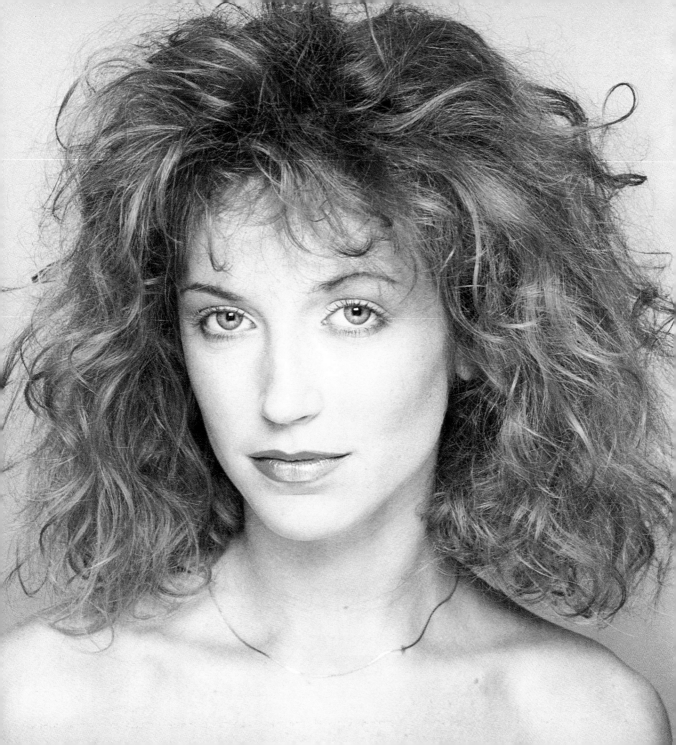

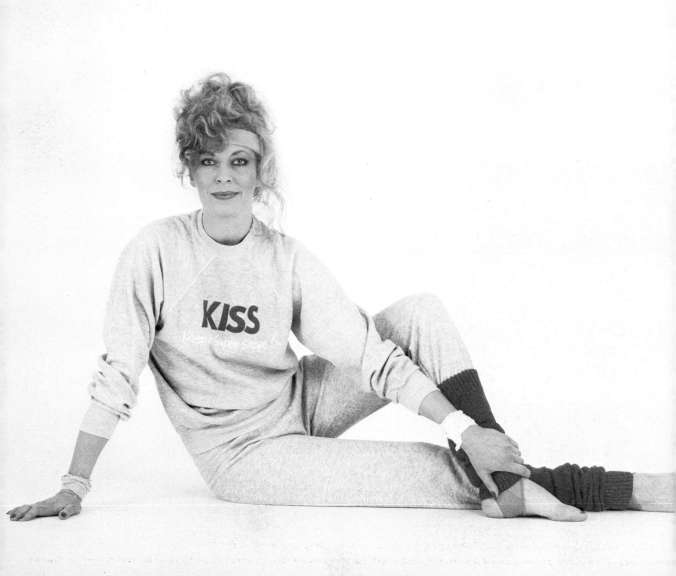

Looking Good

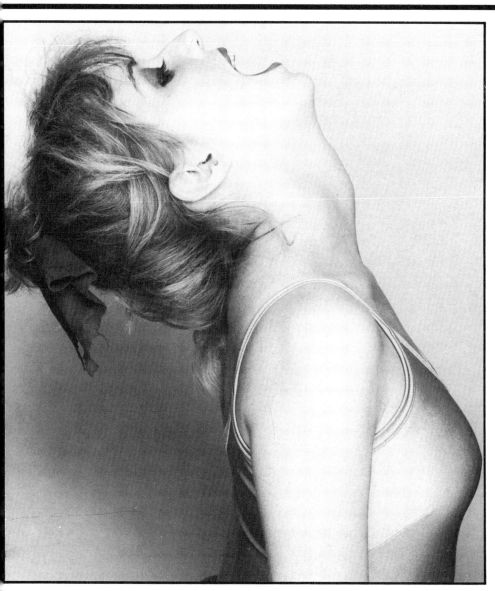

Neck Notes: Your neck and chin need all the help they can get. Drop your head back and have twenty good yawns, once in the morning and again before you go to bed.

Far Left:
Don't you think Gillian looks good in her tracksuit? If you have never worn one before, you are in for a treat; they are comfortable and flattering, too. You'll wonder how you ever did without one!

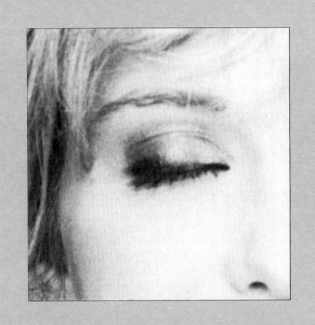

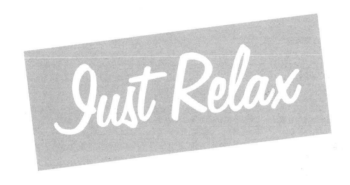

7

Just Relax

Just Relax

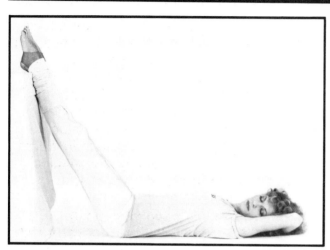

Take it lying down: Lie down and rest your legs on a chair or the edge of the bed; they must be higher than your head. Let everything go very heavy. Your eyes naturally close...

I t sounds like the easiest-ever two-word instruction, but 'just relax' can be impossible if you suffer unresolved stress. That happens when the level of stress in your life gets way out of balance.

Stress is not a dirty word; stress is what can give life its edge of excitement. The trouble starts when the level of stress is wrong for an individual. Think about exams, for instance; they are a stress-stimulator. Some people need that stress to perform well—it keys them up, they feel alert, their memory is sharper than ever before. But for other people, the same stimulation is going to make them fail. For them it brings mental blurring, panic, they feel their heart beating faster, they may sweat profusely, feel sick, and have a dry mouth. In severe cases it may even prove impossible for them to write their name on the paper! But what if the exam was far too easy? That could mean that the stress-stimulator was too low—the candiate just could not be bothered with such a dull, grey task; that, too, could bring failure.

To some extent, you can control the amount of stress in your life, but it tends to go into overdrive in even the best regulated lives. Too much change puts you at risk. It can be sad change like the death of a lover, or good change like going on holiday. Remember, the more changes in your life, the more vulnerable you are to stress. Physical factors can increase the level above that which you can cope with: too much noise, pollution, overcrowding, lack of exercise (see the table).

When the red light goes on, your body reacts by throwing the emergency switch. It's an automatic switch, and one you don't have to think about, which is just as well, when it is an instant physical danger. If a runaway car is about knock you over, there isn't really time to weigh up what the right course of action might be. You automatically jump out of the way. This physical action is just what the body is expecting, just what it needs to switch off the emergency signal and get everything back to normal. In this case the stress is resolved.

But the automatic switch goes on in response to other kinds of strees; stress which won't be resolved by this physical reaction. The pattern is exactly the same: the body prepares itself by releasing three hormones: adrenalin, noradrenalin and cortisol into the bloodstream. The muscles tense; breathing becomes faster and more shallow; heartbeat rises dramatically; lactic acid levels shoot up; great demand is put on the reserves of B and C vitamins.

The body is perfectly prepared to attack or retreat at high speed. The problem is there is no outlet for all that accumulated energy. You could become a victim of an over-stressed life-style (see the next table).

Unresolved stress is dangerous. It is pointless, and harmful, to grit your teeth and ignore the feelings of anxiety and hostility it leaves you with. Better to start the campaign to combat it:

HOW MUCH STRESS IS THERE IN YOUR LIFE?

All of the following are potential stressers:

1. Death of partner	12. Promotion or new job
2. Divorce	13. Premenstrual tension
3. Separation	14. Taking out a large loan
4. Marriage	15. Big personal success
5. Losing job	16. Moving house
6. Getting back together after separation	17. Holidays
	18. Noise
7. Sudden change in health (for better or worse)	19. Poor diet
	20. Pollution
8. Pregnancy	21. Overcrowding
9. Giving up heavy smoking	22. Lack of exercise
10. Sexual problems	23. Boring job
11. Death of close friend	

Your stress tolerance level may be high – but when you know there's extra stress coming into your life it is wise to try the stress resolvers: exercise, diet and relaxation.

SYMPTOMS OF AN OVERSTRESSED LIFE

1. Backache	11. Loss of pleasure in life
2. Breathlessness	12. Overeating
3. Chest pains	13. Pain in neck and shoulders
4. Chronic lateness	14. Palpitations
5. Dizziness	15. Sighing
6. Fainting	16. Sweating for no reason
7. Feelings of isolation	17. Tiredness
8. Headaches	18. Ulcers
9. Heavy smoking	19. Upset stomach
10. Insomnia	

Just Relax

STRESS RESOLVERS
1. Step up your level of exercise, after all it's action that your body has so powerfully prepared for.
2. Go for a very brisk walk or try the aerobercises (but please don't forget the Warm-Up and pulse-rate checks). Use that drive stress is giving you really to work .

FIGHT IT WITH FOOD
In periods of your life when you are susceptible to stress, it is even more vital to check that you're eating properly. Most important of all are the B vitamins, which are actually known as stress-vitamins because they protect the nerves. When your body goes into its stress response, it uses up the Bs very fast; make sure you replace them. Every day you should take up to six Brewer's yeast tablets, and eat wholegrains. When you are under pressure, you are constantly drawing on vitamin C. That will leave you little in reserve to fight off infection and keep cells healthy, unless you monitor your intake and keep it high. Fresh citrus fruits and raw vegetables are a daily must. The nervous system is going to make extra demands on minerals so make sure you keep up calcium supplies by drinking some milk or eating cheese; magnesium supplies may be depleted, so eat a banana at least every other day and keep up zinc by eating wholegrains and seafoods.

DON'T EAT THE STRESS BUILDERS
1. Avoid sugar. It gives a temporary boost but then energy levels tumble making it much more difficult to conquer stress.
2. Stay away from fatty foods, especially high-fat meats like pork and lamb. The minerals so vital to the fight will be diminished.
3. Forget the salt—and that means salty foods like bacon, salted peanuts and crisps. The salt can lead to a draining of potassium. Insufficient potassium in the body can itself set up stress symptoms.
4. Avoid coffee and tea and cola drinks. Look out, too, for hidden caffeine—headache and cold remedies often contain a significantly high dose.

Even with positive action from exercise and diet, there may still be a residue of stress, especially if your lifestyle is exposing you to daily doses. You can tackle that with deep relaxation, to ease away the tensions that are threatening to take permanent hold.

LONG, SLOW RELAXER
Do you know what a relaxed muscle feels like? No, well it's a hard question. The way to identify it is to start with its opposite! Clench your fist really hard until you can see the knuckles grow white. Very gradually let your hand uncurl; go on feeling that relaxation...now you've got it. This is the principle behind deep relaxation. Tense each muscle for six seconds, then spend a minute

Just Relax

or more experiencing it relax and grow heavy. Some people find it helps to repeat the word 'relax', slowly and deliberately.

Choose a comfortable chair or lie on the floor or bed. and go throught the entire sequence:

1. Breathing is the most natural relaxer of all. For a few minutes breathe in to a count of four, out to a count of eight. This will get oxygen really moving round the body helping those muscles to get back to normal.

2. Clench both your fists as tightly as you can. Hold then release very slowly. Concentrate on the sensation of warmth and loosening that's flowing right to the tips of your fingers.

3. Straighten your arms, feel them pull right out of the shoulder sockets, point your fingers hard. Let go. Don't your arms feel heavy?

4. Pull your shoulders up as if you were aiming for your ears. Hold and relax, get them really low, really loose.

5. Screw up your face into a terrific frown. Hold and release.

6. Lift your eyebrows; you are trying to touch your hairline. Hold and release.

7. Bite your teeth together and press your tongue against the roof of your mouth, feel the tension along your jaw. Hold and release. Are you saying the word 'relax' to yourself. Is it helping?

8. Take a very deep breath and feel your chest muscles. Feel them relax as you breathe out again.

9. Pull your stomach right in as if you were trying to make it touch your back. Hold and release.

10. Tighten your bottom so that you are really pulling it together. Hold and release.

11. Straighten your legs, feel them grow longer, point your toes—yes, point really hard! Hold and release.

12. Concentrate on the warmth and heaviness in each of the muscle groups; stay still until thirty minutes is up.

When there isn't time for the long, slow relaxer, try the almost instant relaxing exercise.

SPOT RELAXERS

There is one spot on your body that is the most difficult to relax of all. It may need direct action. That area is your shoulders and the back of your neck.

Shouldering On: This may sound like harsh treatment, but it actually feels very good—though you may get the odd strange look if anyone sees you doing it! It consists just of slapping. Throw your right arm over your left shoulder and slap about fifteen times; repeat with the left arm over the right shoulder. That will warm up the flesh nicely for the next treatment which is pure sensuous pleasure!

THE HOT OIL SHOULDER SOOTHER

This is a simple massage which is even more

Just Relax

effective if you use one of the aromatic oils, or use a few drops of your favourite perfume mixed with mineral oil.

1. Warm a little oil, but don't let it get too hot. Take off your clothes; make sure the room is warm and quiet. For extra tranquility, work by candlelight.

2. Spread oil on the palms of your hands and work gently into the whole of the shoulder and neck area so that your hands can slide smooth and easy over the warm-oiled flesh.

3. Use the palm of your right hand to work on your left shoulder, use firm pressure and press down in circular movements. Work across back stopping just short of spine. If you are not experienced in massage it it best to leave the spine alone. Repeat the pressing movements, but this time using the palm of the left hand on the right shoulder.

4. Starting at the point where the neck meets the shoulders, use your fingertips to slowly rotate the flesh, gradually moving out to the edge of the shoulders.

5. Drop your head forward and fingertip tiny circles from the hairline to the nape of the neck. Make sure there is still enough oil for your fingers to travel smoothly.

6. Use finger and thumb to pinch the flesh everywhere—neck and shoulders—but make it gentle pinches!

7. Clasp hands behind your neck and press down firmly.

8. Finish with very gentle, rhythmic fingertip stroking, starting at the hairline and working down and then out to the edge of your shoulders.

After all of that there should not be even a hint of stress-tension left. But sometimes there is still a sense of uneasiness—and it's probably all in the mind. What you need to do is empty your head of all the busy thoughts that are unproductively jostling around. With all that happening there's not much chance of thinking clearly and objectively. There's little hope of doing any problem solving. What you need is a way of controlling those restless thoughts and releasing the mental tension. Meditation is a sure way of relaxing the mind.

LET THE STRESS FLOAT AWAY

Words, or pictures, or memories—which works best for you? If you're not sure, try all the following techniques:

The Use of Words

1. Sit in your most comfortable chair. The room should be warm and quiet.

2. Find your mantra, the sound that suits you. Experiment with the vowels: a e i o u. Lengthen the sounds; it sometimes helps to put an h on the end so you are saying (like the Bisto kid) ahhhhhhhhhhhhhhhhhhh.

3. When you've found your soul-sound, practise saying it inside your head, and out loud. Stay with the one that feels comfortable.

4. As with the physical relaxation, you should put your breathing into a steady state. Breathe n to the count of four; out to the count of eight.

5. Your mind should be quietening; just the sound matters. Fix on it, block everything else out. Continue for ten minutes.

Picture this

A picture you enjoy looking at, one that makes you feel calm can work just as well as the mantra. Find the picture and prop it up in front of you so that from your most comfortable position—sitting in a chair, or lying down—you can see it without any strain.

Look at the picture intently. At first your thoughts will still jostle, but they will quieten as the picture is taking up the front of your mind. As you become more relaxed you won't need to look intently at the picture; let it go slightly out of focus, and later close your eyes. Stay quiet for ten minutes.

Memory and meditation

If you find the first two methods over-abstract, you can programme your mind with pleasant memories. It could be a walk by the seashore on a summer day, a snowball fight, a romantic dinner. Have a stack of these memories, say half a dozen, on file. When you are feeling particularly tense, forget about the 'here and now' and plug in to those memories. It's just like using the inside of your head as a video.

SLEEP: IT'S THE ONLY WAY TO BE WIDE AWAKE

There is no contradiction in that statement. A good night's sleep is essential for energy, for the good health of every bit of your body. It's while you're peacefully asleep that all the repair and building work goes on.

If you were forced to stay awake for just one night, your reaction time would slow down, memory would be less sharp, and you could feel hostile. Of course, you would be tired; but you could also feel very depressed.

If sleep is good for you, is a lot of sleep better? No. In fact, getting into the habit of sleeping too much makes you feel permanently tired!

Only you can work out what your correct ration of sleep is. Some people thrive on as little as four hours a night; others need ten. Most people settle in at around eight hours. One clue is personality: short-timers are usually extroverts with a high natural rate of physical activity and underneath it all have a rather conservative character. Long-timers are the creative introverts. But they show remarkable stamina and are much less concerned than short-timers about what other people may think of them.

Recognize yourself? The most reliable test for if you've had enough sleep is how you feel when you wake up. If getting out of bed is not too awful, and you feel (at least after a shower) well refreshed, you've found the right level.

Just Relax

There are few things worse than lying in bed feeling exhausted and not being able to get to sleep. It can be a reaction to unresolved stress or may be a symptom of a tired brain in an under-worked body. Exercise will put that right, and the relaxation techniques should help. Try very hard not to take sleeping pills—the quality of sleep you get with their help is never as good as natural sleep. You could try hot milk—the calcium in that is a natural tranquillizer. If you don't like hot milk, try lacing it with a tablespoon of whisky or rum! Still not happy? Take calcium tablets on their own.

Check that you're not eating too late in the evening, and remember that caffeine can keep you awake up to seven hours after you've drunk it if you're particularly susceptible. To be extra safe, don't drink it after lunchtime.

But what if you've done all of that, and you're still not able to sleep?

DON'T JUST LIE THERE

Get out of bed. If you stay in bed when you can't fall asleep, bed will become fixed in your subconscious as a place where you fail to go to sleep. Give yourself thirty minutes to fall asleep. If you're still awake after that, get out of bed and spend about twenty minutes doing some simple physical work, like the washing up, or read a book or listen to some music. Whatever you do, don't even think about sleep.

Go back to bed and give yourself another thirty minutes to fall asleep. If you don't, get up again. Keep repeating the sequence until you do fall asleep. The first few nights you may feel that you're up and down like a bouncing ball. But each night, you'll get up less until the habit of not sleeping has been replaced by the habit of sleeping.

If it's a whirl of thoughts that's keeping you awake, or worry about a challenging day ahead, use the time out of bed to sort it. It sounds over-simple, but it actually does help if you write down on a sheet of paper all the thoughts that are crowding your mind—don't worry if some of them sound trivial. You can make tomorrow look much less forbidding by writing down a plan of exactly what you're going to do from the moment you get up in the morning, with a timetable that will show you how it works.

If your sleeping problems are only slight, it is good to know that one of the oldest, most traditional methods has been shown, by scientific tests, to be one of the most effective ways of nodding off. It is counting, but not sheep, because most of us aren't familiar enough with them to visualise them easily. Best of all is to count backwards from 100, visualising each number in your head as you count it down. Very few people get below 75…

INSTANT RELAXERS

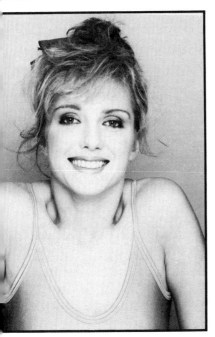
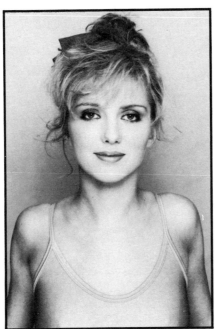
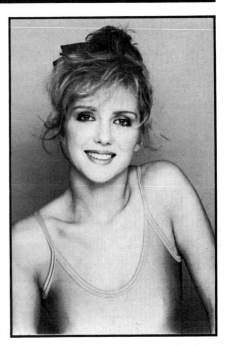

Shoulders to it: Circle the shoulders forward, up, back and down. Do the same in reverse. Raise them really high as if you were going to touch your ears. Go on until you feel the tension work its way out. Then try using one shoulder at a time.

Just Relax

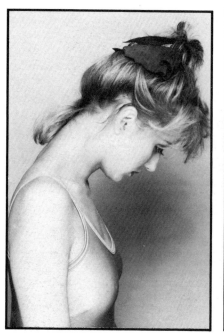 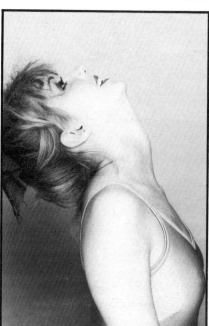 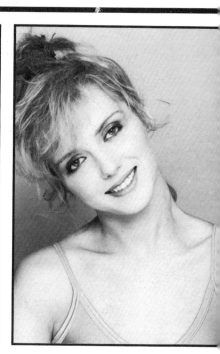

Headfirst: Drop the head forward, up, then back. Now to the right, up and to the left. Then circle it until you feel the tension go.

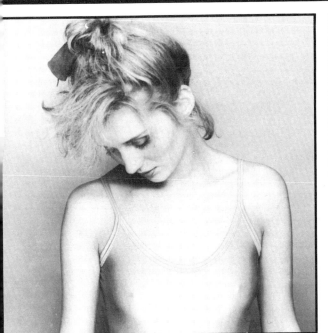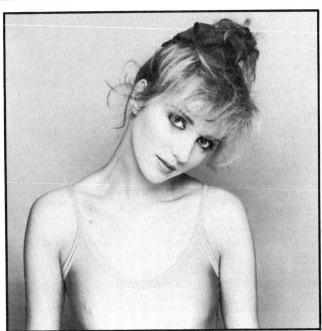

Progress Charts

AEROBERCISES	Now	In 3 months	In 6 months	In 1 year
Resting pulse				
After one minute				
After six minutes				
Times per week				
Duration				

ADVANCED KISS

	Now	In 3 months	In 6 months	In 1 year
Times per week				
Number of Exercises done perfectly				

GENERAL ENERGY LEVEL (tick one)

	Now	In 3 months	In 6 months	In 1 year
Poor				
Fair				
Terrific				

FLEXIBILITY (tick one)

	Now	In 3 months	In 6 months	In 1 year
Poor				
Fair				
Terrific				

STRESS MANAGEMENT (tick one)

	Now	In 3 months	In 6 months	In 1 year
Poor				
Fair				
Good				

Progress Charts

WEIGHT	Now	In 3 months	In 6 months	In 1 year
Ideal				

MEASUREMENTS

Upper arm				
Bust				
Waist				
Hips				
Thighs				
Calves				

FLAB FACTOR (tick one)

Bad				
Going				
Gone				

LEVEL OF EXERCISE

Warm Up Times per week				
Number of Exercises done perfectly				

KISS

Times per week				
Number of Exercises done perfectly				